SHADOWS

A HISTORY OF THE OLMSTED MEDICAL CENTER

G. RICHARD GEIER, JR., MD

Printed in the United States of America

5 4 3 2 1

Library of Congress Control Number: 2010923418

ISBN 13: 978-0-615-35457-6
ISBN 10: 0-615-35457-2

Contents

Part I: In the Shadow

Chapter 1. Before the Beginning

Chapter 2. Dr. Wente and the Olmsted Medical Group

Chapter 3. A Community Hospital at Last

Chapter 4. Boom Times

Chapter 5. Change and Opportunities

Chapter 6. Troubled Times at the Olmsted Community Hospital

Chapter 7. Troubled Times at the Olmsted Medical Group

Part II: Out of the Shadow

Chapter 8. Changing of the Guard

Chapter 9. New Structures

Chapter 10. The Olmsted Medical Center

Chapter 11. Into the New Millennium

Chapter 12. Looking Back, and Forward

Appendix A. Roster of Olmsted Medical Group and Olmsted Medical Center Physicians, Podiatrists, and Psychologists

Index of Names

General Index

Foreword

Why do we care about history? We've all heard the old saw about how those who don't know history are condemned to repeat it. But I think the most important reason to study history is to help us answer such fundamental existential questions as "Who are we? What are we? Where did we come from?" and "How did we get to be what we are?" Peters and Waterman, in their best-selling book on management, *In Search of Excellence*, talked about developing an organizational mythology, an explanation of how things came to be. Collins and Porras, in *Built to Last*, emphasized the importance of lasting core values in the ability of organizations to succeed over generations. It is in this spirit that this volume was produced, to describe the past of the Olmsted Medical Center for the benefit of its present and future staff, patients, and friends.

In his Preface to *The Gathering Storm*, Churchill stated that he followed the method of Defoe's *Memoirs of a Cavalier*, in which the author hangs the chronicle and discussion of great events on the personal experiences of an individual. Referring to this, Ashley, in *Churchill as Historian*, notes that Churchill often started with a researched historical background, then moved into his own experience, melding history with memoir. This semi-personal history of the Olmsted Medical Center is in much the same form, if on a less grandiose scale. There are disadvantages, of course, to having history written by a participant. Churchill famously stated on several occasions things like, "It will be up to history to judge. Of course, I intend to write the history." When he began writing his *History of the Second World War*, he was his party's leader in Parliament and by the latter volumes was prime minister. What he wrote had to be tempered by domestic and international politics, respect for friends' reputations, and concern for libel suits. I'm not too concerned about the effects of this volume on international relations, but I don't have the freedom of expression that a later historian would have. Still, there are advantages in knowing more than is preserved in minutes and other documents, particularly when many documents are missing and many minutes are so brief as to be useless to one who was not there.

It has long been considered remarkable that one of the world's leading medical centers could have grown up in a small town in rural Minnesota. It is no less remarkable that a leading community medical center could later grow up in the same place.

1

This history is more doctor-centric than I would have liked. This is largely due to the loss of nearly all the hospital board minutes; it is also due to the volume of material that I have saved and to Dr. Harold Wente's sharing his memoirs and collected papers, the great majority of both relating to the Olmsted Medical Group. The historian H.W. Van Loon said, "The history of the world is the record of a man in quest of his daily bread and butter." That is, it's about more than kings and generals. The story of the Olmsted Medical Center, too, is much more than that of the doctors. It is the story of Jim Cannady, one of the original hospital orderlies, who became an LPN, RN, purchasing director, and interim administrator. It's about Rita Cunningham, a radiology technician, and her brother Kevin, a nurse anesthetist, who served hospital patients for a combined 81 years. It's about thousands of people doing hundreds of jobs and about tens of thousands of patients. Unfortunately, I can't tell all their stories, but I can try to show the development of the organization and its mission, vision, and core values.

It can also serve as a resource for the future author of the centennial history and as a stimulus for establishing a useful archive to prevent losses of future historical material. Minnesota Public Radio's morning show had a fictitious sponsor, The Future Historians of America, whose motto was "Preparing for tomorrow's yesterdays today." It was meant as comedy, but I think it is really a good idea. We need not only to learn how we came to be, but also to help our successors learn how they will have come to be.

Acknowledgments

First, I must mention two sources that could be considered co-authors. One is Nora H. Guthrey, Dr. Will Mayo's private secretary from 1919 until his death in 1939. Ms. Guthrey authored a series of papers on the history of medicine prior to 1900 in Houston and Fillmore counties that was published in *Minnesota Medicine* from 1945 to 1949. She then wrote a longer paper titled, "Medicine and its Practitioners in Olmsted County Prior to 1900," which ran serially each month from July 1949 through September 1951. The early part of Chapter 1 of *Shadows* draws heavily from this work. The other is Dr. Harold A. Wente, the founder of the Olmsted Medical Group, who, after retiring, wrote his memoirs for his family and a few favored friends, of whom I am grateful to be one. These, along with a few visits and innumerable phone calls, are the basis for most of Chapter 2 and much of Chapters 4 and 5. I acknowledge these two sources here and have avoided a plethora of quotation marks, brackets, and ellipses in the text for ease of reading.

I have had assistance finding materials from a number of individuals. The ladies of the Olmsted Community Hospital Auxiliary, especially the late Julia Bohmbach, kept yearly scrapbooks of dated newspaper clippings and other memorabilia, which saved me many tedious hours of poring over microfilmed newspaper archives. Nicole Babcock of the Mayo Foundation Historical Section furnished the William F. Braasch papers and other bits of information. Marilyn Helmsley, assistant librarian at the History Center of Olmsted County, informed me of Guthrey's work and provided a wealth of other information. Richard Devlin, the Olmsted County administrator, and his assistants, Suzanne LaPalm and Sally Trom, provided Olmsted county board minutes, and Mary Wellick and Sherry Haugen of the Olmsted County Public Health department provided minutes of the health board and the community health center board. Nancy King of S&S Moving and Storage and Sharon Strum of the Olmsted Medical Center helped in my unsuccessful search for the Olmsted Community Hospital board minutes. Sue Graves-Johnson, Joel Messmer, and Larry Udstuen of the Olmsted Medical Center, Joel Rueber and Alan Fleischmann of the Mayo Clinic, Donald Fisher and his staff at the American Medical Group Association, and Angela Curran of the Center for the History of Family Medicine also provided useful information. Gretchen Merideth of the Rochester *Post-Bulletin* was helpful in identifying and providing photographs, as was the History Center of Olmsted County.

Finally, I am grateful to Dr. David Westgard, Tim Weir, Stacey Vanden Heuvel and, especially, Dr. Roy Yawn for their review of the text and for helpful suggestions. My editor, Jennifer Gangloff, was extremely helpful and made the book much better than it would have been. I did not take all her suggestions, though, so don't blame her for any deficiencies. Jeremy Salucka and Wes Duellman of the OMC Regional Foundation staff were helpful in the publication of the book.

Part I: In the Shadow

"Family Practice in the Shadow of the Mayo Clinic"

Headline, *Medical Economics*, August 17, 1959, p. 90.

Chapter 1
Before the Beginning

The need for the Olmsted Medical Center arose from the unusual history of medicine in Rochester and Olmsted County reaching back almost to the county's beginning. The influence of the Mayo Clinic on local medical practice was to play a significant role in the origin, growth, and development of the medical center and its hospital.

When the Minnesota territory was formed in 1849, the future site of Rochester was beyond the frontier. There were only a few hundred Europeans in Minnesota along the rivers that had brought them, the Mississippi, Minnesota, and St. Croix. In the summer of 1851, the treaties of Mendota and Traverse de Sioux opened large areas of Minnesota to settlement, and settlers flooded into the state by the tens of thousands, pushing westward from the rivers, across the woods and prairies, establishing farms and towns and businesses. One of the first settlers to arrive in what would become Olmsted County was a physician, Dr. John L. Balcombe, who in 1852 led a small band of explorers from La Crosse, Wisconsin, along the high ground between the Zumbro and Root rivers into the future High Forest Township. There he claimed a parcel of forested land, which he later sold and which became the site of High Forest village.[1] The frontier reached what was to become Rochester in the spring of 1854, when Thomas C. Cummings and Robert McReady built shanties near Cascade Creek. In July 1854 George Head settled on the Zumbro River in what is now downtown Rochester.[2] Another 1854 arrival was Joseph Alexander, an herbalist who sometimes used the title of doctor. He had an extensive practice which was continued by his daughter after his death in 1896.[3] Olmsted County was carved out of the western parts of Wabasha and Winona counties in 1855.[4] The county seat was established in 1857 at Rochester, which had been platted[5] in 1855.

---

[1]   Later that year, Dr. Balcombe became one of the first settlers of Winona, where he died in 1856. Curtis-Wedge, Franklin. *History of Winona County.* Chicago: H.C. Cooper, Jr. & Co., 1913. pp. 128-144.

[2]   *History of Winona, Olmsted and Dodge Counties.* Chicago: H.H. Hill & Co., 1884. pp. 623-624.

[3]   The medical history to 1900 in this chapter is drawn from Guthrey unless otherwise noted.

[4]   *History of Wabasha and Winona Counties.* Chicago: H.H. Hill & Co., 1884. p. 598.

[5]   The town site was surveyed, streets laid out, and lots defined.

A number of medical practitioners of various sorts were among the early settlers in southeast Minnesota. The most notable were Dr. Hector Galloway, Dr. Ira C. Bardwell, Dr. Lewis Kelley, Dr. Edwin Childs Cross, Dr. Elisha Wild Cross, and Dr. William Worrall Mayo, the father of two sons who later founded the Mayo Clinic.

The first regular physician[6] to settle in Olmsted County was Dr. Hector Galloway, who arrived in Oronoco in 1855. Dr. Galloway was born in Cattaraugus County, New York, on June 28, 1828. When he was eighteen, he began teaching school during the winter and studying medicine the rest of the year. He entered Geneva Medical College in New York in 1852, graduating after the required two courses of lectures. He first moved west to practice in McGregor, Iowa. He then moved to Oronoco, Minnesota, where he spent nine years, and then to Rochester, where he became a leader of the young medical community. Dr. Galloway moved to Fargo, North Dakota, in 1879, then to Tacoma, Washington, before returning to Rochester in 1894. He died on March 4, 1899, at his brother's home in Otto, New York.

Early in 1856, Dr. Ira C. Bardwell, a respected physician and surgeon, arrived in Rochester. Born in Wayne County, New York, in 1812, he grew up in nearby Livingston County, where he read medicine[7] in the office of a Dr. Champlaine. He then studied and attended medical lectures for two years in Willoughby, Ohio, before working his way west practicing medicine. In 1859, he moved with his family from Rochester to the nearby prosperous village of Pleasant Grove, where he practiced for many years.

Dr. Lewis Kelley (1808-1872) practiced in Rochester from 1857 to 1863. He left a permanent mark on Rochester by building in 1858 the city's first brick building, a two-story structure of locally kilned bricks, which still stands on the northeast corner of Broadway and Fourth Street Southeast.[8] His office was in front, and his family lived in the rear of the building. They also owned the city's first piano, a novel source of entertainment in the frontier community. Dr. Kelley rented the second floor to a newspaper, the *Rochester City Post*. He went into the newspaper publishing business

---

[6]   As opposed to "irregular" or unscientific practitioners.
[7]   In this era would-be doctors and lawyers often read professional books in the office of a practitioner and acted as something like apprentices for a period of months, rarely more than a year, before beginning practice.
[8]   This was the south end of Broadway, which extended only two blocks northward.

himself in 1860, first in Rochester and then moving to Owatonna, Northfield, and Faribault.[9]

Dr. Edwin Childs Cross, one of the earliest and best educated of the pioneer physicians and surgeons of Olmsted County, came to Rochester in May 1858 from Brattleboro, Vermont. Born in 1824 at Bradford, Vermont, Dr. Cross graduated from Dartmouth College. He studied medicine at several colleges before receiving a medical degree from Norwich University in Vermont in 1846. After the death of their first child and the loss of their home by fire a few weeks later, he and his wife set out for Minnesota. His younger brother, Dr. Elisha Wild Cross, had visited Rochester two years earlier in 1856, and on his return east, had described the growing community and its need for physicians. While there were several physicians living in Rochester in 1858, it appears that only Dr. Bardwell was practicing, and even he moved on the following year. By 1860, the elder Dr. Cross had become so well established that he sent for his brother to join him in practice. Their partnership was interrupted when Dr. Elisha Cross was appointed assistant surgeon of the Fourth Regiment, Minnesota Volunteer Infantry, in December 1861. He served throughout the Civil War with the western army under generals Grant and Sherman. After the war, the brothers practiced separately, but in close association.

Dr. William Worrall Mayo was born near Manchester, England, May 31, 1819. Despite his father's death when William was only seven, he had a better-than-average education, including some time at the Pine Street Medical School in Manchester, tutelage by the famous scientist John Dalton, and some rudimentary medical training in London and Glasgow. A lifelong wanderer,[10] W.W. Mayo took ship for New York in 1845. After a stint working in the drug room[11] at Bellevue Hospital, he continued west via a well-established migration route through Buffalo, the Great Lakes, and down into Indiana. After a partnership in a tailor shop in Lafayette, Indiana, he returned to studying medicine under Dr. Elizur Deming. He graduated from Indiana Medical College in La Porte in 1850 and returned to Lafayette, where he married, and practiced briefly in partnership with

---

[9]   Dr. Kelley died in Owatonna in 1872 and is buried in Oakwood Cemetery in Rochester.

[10]   Mayo, C.W. *Mayo: the Story of my Family and my Career,* p. 5. Garden City, N.Y.: Doubleday, 1968.

[11]   The predecessor to a hospital inpatient pharmacy.

Dr. Deming. He moved to St. Louis, Missouri, in the fall of 1853, where he received a doctor of medicine degree the next spring from the University of Missouri. Dr. Mayo then moved to St. Paul, Minnesota, where he explored the wilderness while his wife ran a millinery shop as she had in Lafayette. In 1856, he moved his family near Le Sueur, where he farmed and practiced medicine part time. They moved into Le Sueur itself in 1859, where Dr. Mayo published a newspaper and worked on riverboats in addition to maintaining his practice. When the military draft for the Civil War started in 1862, Dr. Mayo became the examining surgeon[12] for Le Sueur County. Shortly after he assumed this position, the Sioux Uprising of 1862 broke out. Dr. Mayo was one of three physicians who marched to New Ulm with an improvised militia and cared for casualties during the ensuing battle. In April 1863, he was named examiner of the military enrollment board for the first Minnesota congressional district, headquartered in Rochester, and was assisted by Dr. Galloway. Dr. Mayo moved to Rochester immediately, and his family followed the next January. In early 1865, Dr. Mayo was replaced as examiner by Dr. Edwin C. Cross but Dr. Mayo had started a medical practice in his spare time, and had built a comfortable house, and he finally stayed put. His grandson, Dr. Charles W. "Chuck" Mayo wrote, "… the main reason Grandfather allowed his family to root in Rochester was that Grandmother finally put her foot down and told him she would wander no more."[13]

Dr. Hector Galloway, Dr. Edwin Cross, Dr. Elisha Cross, and Dr. William W. Mayo were typical of the better frontier doctors of their generation. As well educated as possible by the standards of the time, they were driven westward to see what was beyond, often holding public offices or working at other jobs, as medicine paid too poorly to support a family. They also farmed much of the time, as did most other folk. All four were founders of the Olmsted County Medical Society. In addition to being a leader in spreading scientific medicine to the frontier, Dr. Mayo participated in the reorganization of the Minnesota State Medical Association and served as its president in 1873. He also served as mayor of Rochester (1882-1883). Dr. Galloway served on the Rochester Board of Health and Board of Education and as county coroner, and was elected to the State Senate. Dr. Edwin Cross was another leader of the profession for more than three decades. He was active in the Minnesota State Medical Association and was a delegate to the American Medical

---

[12] A physician contracted by the army to examine recruits for their fitness to serve.
[13] Mayo, C.W., p. 10.

Association. He served several terms on the Rochester Board of Health and was a preceptor[14] for medical students for more than 20 years. Like Dr. Mayo, Dr. Elisha Cross traveled widely to enhance his education, and had a record of public service similar to his brother's. He served on the Minnesota State Board of Health as well. When he died, Dr. Christopher Graham was a pallbearer, and Dr. Will Mayo drafted the Medical Society's tribute.

Dr. Edwin Cross and Dr. William W. Mayo both farmed east of Rochester and raised improved hybrid breeds of cattle and sheep. They shared a love of fast, spirited horses and were known as daredevils driving them with their buggies, but they sometimes paid the price. Dr. Mayo once lost control of his team, which smashed the buggy into a tree, stunning him and bloodying his nose.[15] Dr. Cross was less fortunate. On July 4, 1894, his team was spooked by firecrackers thrown into the street, and the horses bolted. His carriage crashed into a tree, throwing the doctor out onto a picket fence. He died the following day.[16]

In the last half of the nineteenth century, especially from the end of the Civil War until 1883, Minnesota was a hotbed for all sorts of irregular practitioners, mainly itinerant, and many from Illinois and Wisconsin, which had passed regulatory laws that forced them to seek patients elsewhere. There were the almost-respectable homeopaths, followers of Samuel Hahnemann (1755-1843), a German doctor who treated patients with highly diluted doses of substances that were thought to produce in healthy people symptoms similar to the disease they were treating. There were also eclectic, electric, and magnetic healers, using imaginative or imaginary technology. One such "cured" arthritis by means of "renowned European chains." Another had "peculiar natural and healing powers," attributed to his being the seventh son of a seventh son. There were medicine shows such as the Wizard Oil Troupe and the Kickapoo Medical Company that visited Rochester. These provided concerts and other entertainment while hawking their cure-all tonics, which were mostly alcohol. The newspapers railed against "tramp doctors" but also advertised all the tonics and at least eleven brands of "bitters," which were alcoholic preparations of herbs, barks and roots, alleged to assist digestion. Pushed by the state medical association to restrain these irregular practitioners, Minnesota passed its first medical licensing law in 1883, but

---

[14] A physician in whose offices students "read medicine."
[15] Clapesattle, H. *The Doctors Mayo*. Minneapolis: University of Minnesota Press, 1941, p. 114.
[16] Guthrey, N.H.

homeopaths were included and the other existing irregular practitioners were exempt from licensing requirements for five years.

The Drs. Cross, William W. Mayo, and Galloway were also the physicians of Olmsted County who performed the greatest number of surgical operations, often assisting each other in various combinations. Operations were mostly for trauma, abscesses, and amputations. Antisepsis had not yet arrived, much less asepsis.[17] From December 1876 until June 1878, Dr. Elisha Cross and Dr. William W. Mayo were partners, sharing offices over Geisinger and Newton's drugstore on Broadway. In the years before there were local hospitals, patients were usually operated upon in their own homes. By the 1870s, Rochester surgeons had begun to use rooms in local hotels for operating rooms and postoperative care of patients from out of town. Beginning in the 1880s, Dr. Mayo had a small hospital of eight or nine beds for several years in the home of a practical nurse at Broadway and Seventh Street Northwest, later the site of the original Samaritan Bethany nursing home. He also used rooms in some of the smaller hotels to treat transients.

Probably Dr. William W. Mayo's greatest contribution to medicine was raising his sons to become physicians and seeing that they were as well educated as possible. The entrance of Dr. William J. "Will" Mayo into practice in 1883 after he graduated from the University of Michigan brought new operations in areas of elective[18] surgery, as well as the first application of Listerism, or antisepsis. The return of Dr. Charles H. "Charlie" Mayo in 1888, fresh from the Chicago Medical College of Northwestern University, brought still more new procedures, including surgery for the thyroid. All this, despite the fact that neither Dr. Will nor Dr. Charlie had had any surgical training, not even an internship after medical school.

Meanwhile, in January 1879, the second Minnesota Hospital for the Insane opened in Rochester. This brought a new group of physicians to the community, who joined the county medical society and stimulated an interest in psychiatric and nervous disorders among the general practitioners. The hospital was renamed the Rochester State Hospital in 1893.

---

[17] Antisepsis, or Listerism, used antiseptics, mainly carbolic acid, to kill germs to try to prevent infection. Asepsis came soon afterwards and uses modern sterile techniques to avoid getting germs into wounds.
[18] Non-emergency.

A defining event in Rochester's history was the tornado that struck the city on August 21, 1883. The improbable outcome of this disaster would be the transformation of Rochester from an anonymous little farm town into a leading medical center of the world. The tornado killed sixteen people within the city and five more in surrounding areas. Forty-one were injured, including one of the town's doctors. Many more were made homeless.[19] The city council asked Dr. W.W. Mayo to take charge of the injured, which he did, assisted by all the other doctors in town. He sent for the Sisters of St. Francis, a newly established order of teachers, to help with the nursing. Mother Alfred Moes, on seeing the scope of the disaster, offered the use of the larger convent[20] to house one hundred of the victims, but it was soon overwhelmed with injured and homeless, so the care of the wounded was transferred the next day to Rommel's Dance Hall at Broadway and Center Street. This makeshift facility convinced Mother Alfred that Rochester needed a permanent hospital. She suggested the idea of a hospital to Dr. W.W. Mayo, but he initially thought that it was not financially feasible. She persisted, however, and said that if Dr. Mayo would promise to take charge of a hospital, the sisters would finance it. It took Mother Alfred four years to raise the funds. On July 26, 1887, the congregation of Our Lady of Lourdes of the Sisters of St. Francis voted to build the hospital, and four months later the sisters paid $2,200 in cash for nine acres just west of town on Zumbro Street (now Second Street Southwest). Drs. W.W. and Will Mayo made a trip east to study the latest in hospital design. Construction contracts were signed August 1, 1888, for a 45-bed hospital with an operating room, and building began soon after.[21] The sisters planned to begin receiving patients on October 1, 1889, but the Mayos had scheduled an eye operation on the preceding day and the operating room was ready, so St. Marys Hospital opened a day early.[22, 23]

The hospital was not intended to be solely for the use of the Mayos, but anti-Catholic prejudice kept other physicians from joining the staff. At the same time, not all the sisters supported expanding their mission from strictly teaching, and many Catholics in the community objected to having Protestant physicians working in what was considered the Catholic hospital. This was the heyday of the American Protective Association, an anti-immigrant and

---

[19] *History of Winona, Olmsted and Dodge Counties.* Chicago: H.H. Hill & Co., 1884. p. 763.
[20] Located on Center Street between Sixth and Seventh Avenues Southwest.
[21] Mayo, C.W., pp. 17-20.
[22] Clapesattle, H., p. 252.
[23] Whelan, Sister Ellen. *The Sisters' Story.* Rochester: Mayo Foundation, pp. 41-49.

anti-Catholic group founded in Clinton, Iowa, in 1887, and active through the 1890s. Sectarian feelings ran high.[24, 25, 26] Gradually, some of the other Rochester physicians began to use St. Marys, but mainly as a pesthouse for patients with dangerous infections and for dying patients. As the hospital's mortality rate began to climb, the sisters in 1891 decided that no patient should be admitted without first being examined by or referred to the Mayos. The effect was that St. Marys became a closed staff hospital open only to the Mayos and their partners,[27] with long-lasting effects on the community.

Rochester doctors not associated with the Mayos did not have unrestricted use of any hospital until another hospital was established in 1892 by Dr. Wilson A. Allen (1834-1934). Dr. Allen "read medicine" for five years in his native Indiana, then being in poor health, he came to Plainview, Minnesota, in 1865 for the healthier climate. In September 1872, he moved to Rochester, where he purchased a homeopathic practice. He eventually received a degree from the homeopathic Hahnemann Medical College in Chicago. In the spring of 1892, he took a partner, Dr. Charles T. Granger (1870-1939), a Rochester native, a former student of his, and a recent Hahnemann graduate. In November 1892, they opened the Riverside Hospital on the east side of the Zumbro River at 134 Line Street (Fifth Street Southeast),[28] about where the north end of the old lumber shed next to the former Fullerton Lumber building stands, in the current Mayo Clinic remote parking lot off Third Avenue Southeast. The building had been a large residence and was remodeled and equipped as a hospital, modern for its time and employing a competent nursing staff. This hospital was open to all physicians and was used by many of the Protestant doctors, but the Mayos continued to keep all their patients at St. Marys. In September 1895, though, the Riverside Hospital suddenly closed without explanation, and Dr. Allen moved his practice to St. Paul in partnership with Dr. O.H. Hall. He maintained a home in Rochester and continued to serve as mayor, a position he held from 1895 through 1896. Early in 1896, he terminated his practice in St. Paul and returned home for good, where he practiced for many years, dying at age 100, a popular and widely respected citizen.[29]

---

[24] Whelan, E., pp. 71-3.
[25] Clapesattle, H., pp. 264-5.
[26] Protestant Paranoia: The American Protective Association Oath. http://historymatters.gmu.edu/d/5351/
[27] Clapesattle, H., pp. 263-4.
[28] *Rochester Post*, Nov. 11, 1892, p. 3.
[29] Clapesattle ends this story with the "astonishing" closing of the hospital and Dr. Allen's

Starting in the summer of 1896, Dr. Granger practiced alone for eight years. In 1898, he married Katherine Cornelie, who had been the supervisor of nurses at the Riverside Hospital. The Rochester Post and Record reported on June 24, 1904, that Dr. Granger had "probably the largest individual practice of any physician outside the Mayos." He served on the city council from 1900 to 1905 and was president of the Olmsted County Medical Society in 1906. In 1904, Dr. Granger took into partnership one of his former students, Dr. George T. Joyce, who had graduated with a degree in medicine from the University of Illinois and, like himself, was a native of Olmsted County. Dr. Granger was credited with making the first diagnoses of infantile paralysis, Spanish flu, and pellagra in Minnesota, and with diagnosing the first case of trichinosis in Rochester. In 1928, he and his wife moved to McGregor, Minnesota. After his wife died there, he returned to Rochester in 1930, but failing health limited his practice, and Dr. Granger died on October 4, 1939.

The closing of Riverside left the Mayos in control of the only hospital in a large area and with a unique and growing surgical practice. By 1900, they had added five partners, Drs. Augustus W. Stinchfield, Christopher Graham (Dr. Charlie's brother-in-law), Gertrude Booker Granger (Dr. Granger's sister-in-law), Melvin C. Millett, and Isabella Herb. At the time, ten other physicians were listed in the City Directory, along with one magnetic healer.[30] In the early twentieth century, hospitals were not yet important for most physicians, as demonstrated by Dr. Granger's success. Instead, patients were typically cared for in their own homes or in convalescent homes. Only major surgery required the use of a hospital, and many of the hospitals of the time were not much more than a hotel or nursing home and often were converted private residences. Even the Mayo Clinic had no dedicated beds for the use of its internal medicine physicians until 1920. The chance discovery of X-rays by Wilhelm Conrad von Roentgen in November 1895 revolutionized diagnostic medicine. By early the next summer, Dr. J.A. Grosvenor Cross (1870-1928), the youngest child of Dr. Edwin C. Cross, assembled a workable X-ray machine in Rochester and produced a successful picture of his wife's hand after a three-hour exposure. In August 1896, he showed the first diagnostic X-ray pictures in the area

---

"hasty departure." The hospital may have failed financially in the depression following the panic of 1893, or Dr. Allen may have simply been overwhelmed by his work. In contrast, only the dedication of the nuns kept St. Marys going in the early years.
[30] *Rochester City and Olmsted County Directory 1900*. The Minnesota Directory Company, Albert Lea.

at the Southern Minnesota Medical Society meeting. Dr. Cross produced diagnostic X-rays for the Mayos until 1900, when they obtained a machine of their own. In 1902, Dr. Cross sold his practice to study in Europe, and then returned to Minneapolis, where he practiced internal medicine until his death on March 3, 1928, after an automobile crash.[31, 32]

As the Mayos' needs grew faster than St. Marys could expand, they began to use additional facilities reserved exclusively for them. In 1906, they used a part of John Kahler's Cook House hotel until he built the Kahler House in 1907. Also in 1906, Charles Chute built the Chute Sanitorium at 123 West Third Street. The next year, he opened a large addition including an operating room for the Mayos and their partners. In 1912, the Mayos again took over a floor of the Cook House, this time for orthopedic surgery. In 1915, Mr. Kahler opened the Colonial Hospital. The Stanley, Worrall, Curie, and Olmsted[33] hospitals were opened by 1920, the first temporarily housing internal medicine.[34, 35] There were other non-hospital facilities in town, too. The Cascade Rest and Milk Sanitarium was opened in 1918 by Dr. John E. Crewe (1872-1947), who had purchased Dr. Grosvenor Cross' practice and who served as Olmsted County coroner from 1911 to 1946. After the Mayos no longer needed the Chute Sanitorium, it was sold and continued in operation until 1917. In 1922, the Samaritan Convalescent Hospital and Hotel opened on the northwest corner of Broadway and Seventh Street Northwest in a modern brick building, sponsored by the Evangelical Church of Peace (now Peace United Church of Christ). It later became the Samaritan Bethany nursing home and was demolished in 1992.

After the First World War, modern medicine increasingly required hospital facilities but the Mayo Clinic[36] had exclusive use of all the hospitals in Rochester, making the city and nearby towns unattractive for independent physicians. By the end of the Second World War, the Mayo Clinic had grown

---

[31] Guthrey, N.H. This is the end of Guthrey's contribution.

[32] Dr. J.A. Grosvenor Cross is buried with his father at Oakwood Cemetery.

[33] No relation to Olmsted Community Hospital.

[34] Clapesattle, H., pp. 500-608.

[35] All the surviving hospitals except St. Marys were replaced by Rochester Methodist Hospital, which opened in October 1960.

[36] The name Mayo Clinic was gradually imposed by visiting physicians. It appears in the city directory for the first time in the 1915-1916 edition.

to 198 physicians[37] while the number of practicing non-Mayo Clinic doctors had shrunk to two in Rochester and one each in Stewartville and Eyota. Efforts to recruit additional general practitioners had failed due to the lack of a hospital for them to use.[38]

* * *

There had been some interest among Rochester's business community at least as early as 1937 in establishing a hospital for non-Mayo Clinic physicians and their patients.[39] Dr. William F. Braasch,[40] the prominent long-time head of the Mayo Clinic section of urology, was a next-door neighbor of Dr. Crewe[41] and had had conversations with him through the years about the problems of practicing without a hospital. Dr. Braasch's father-in-law was Dr. Augustus W. Stinchfield, who had been in general practice in Eyota before becoming the Mayos' first partner. As a member of the board of trustees of the American Medical Association, Dr. Braasch had also become aware of the problems of general practitioners nationally. Upon his retirement in 1946, Dr. Braasch, with the encouragement of Olmsted County Board Commissioner C.B. Vihstadt, took up the cause of a community hospital. On January 15, 1947, he met with a group of independent physicians from Olmsted and surrounding counties at the Carlton Hotel to discuss the idea of a new hospital. They all expressed support.[42, 43] At the same time, the county health department decided to build a new community health center, and a committee had been created to develop the plan.[44] At a Board of Health and Welfare meeting that same January evening the physicians met, Dr. F.M. Feldman, the county health officer, reported that the physicians supported the idea of a new hospital and that Dr. Braasch was willing to help with the health center project.

---

[37] *Rochester City and Olmsted County, Minnesota Directory 1945-1946*. Rochester, Minnesota: Keiter Directory Co.

[38] *Rochester Post-Bulletin*, Sep. 11, 1948.

[39] *Rochester Post-Bulletin*, Oct. 29, 1948, p. 22.

[40] Pronounced Brash, not Brahsh.

[41] Dr. Crewe lived at 801 Third Street, SW, diagonally across the street from the back of Dr. Will Mayo's property. Dr. Braasch was at 815 on the narrow dead-end lane near St. Marys.

[42] William F. Braasch papers, Mayo Foundation Historical Unit.

[43] Olmsted County Board of Health and Welfare Minutes, Jan. 22, 1947.

[44] Olmsted County Board of Health and Welfare Minutes, Dec. 20, 1946.

A week earlier, at a meeting of the Health Center Building Committee, Mr. A.J. Lobb, a Mayo Clinic administrator and committee member, had stated that a major problem for the Mayo Clinic was the hospital situation in Rochester that had led to a decrease in the number of local practicing physicians. The Mayo Clinic felt that this was not desirable and was not its wish. Physicians would not come to Rochester without a hospital in which to practice. Mr. Lobb pointed out that two-thirds of Mayo Clinic patients came from out of state and that Mayo Clinic's hospitals were highly specialized and inappropriate for local private practitioners. Dr. Feldman then suggested that Mayo Clinic organize a section on local practice instead. Mr. Lobb said that such a plan had been discussed by some of the Mayo Clinic staff, but that the Mayo Clinic considered that plan impractical.[45]

Dr. Braasch met with the Board of Health and Welfare on February 4. He discussed the need for a community hospital and the advantages of combining it with the proposed health center, including the sharing of laboratory and radiology facilities. The need for such combined institutions was recognized in the recently passed Hill-Burton Act, which would provide federal funding for up to one-third of the construction cost.[46]

Dr. Braasch then organized the Citizens' Voluntary Hospital Committee, with Leonard Eckstrand, the manager of the local Woolworth's store, as chairman. The Minnesota Board of Health supported the need for the hospital, and the committee members elicited support from various community organizations.[47] On November 10, 1947, Dr. Braasch and Avery Tews, the mayor of Stewartville, whose efforts to recruit physicians to his town had been unsuccessful three separate times because of the lack of a hospital for them,[48] met with the Olmsted County Board. The board then scheduled a special meeting for January 9, 1948, to consider a $500,000 bond issue to finance a hospital. The hospital would be built next to the health department at Fourth Street and Sixth Avenue Southeast on the east side of Bear Creek on land provided at no cost by the Rochester public utility department.[49] At the special meeting, Dr. Braasch urged immediate action, pointing out that "… the sooner the bond issue is approved, the

---

45 Committee on Health Center Building Minutes, Jan. 15, 1947.
46 William F. Braasch papers, Mayo Foundation Historical Unit.
47 *Rochester Post-Bulletin*, Nov. 5, 1947, p. 15.
48 *Rochester Post-Bulletin*, Sep. 11, 1948.
49 Olmsted County Board Minutes, Nov. 10, 1947.

better the chance this county will have to obtain federal funds for part of the expense of building the community hospital."[50] Commissioner Vihstadt then moved that the question of the issuance of bonds at a higher amount of $600,000 be submitted to the voters of Olmsted County at an election to be held on March 9, 1948, for building a county hospital. This motion was defeated three to two; the majority favored waiting until the fall general election for the referendum rather than holding a special vote.[51]

The county board approved employing Mr. T.G. Evenson and Associates, Inc. as the bond consulting firm "if a bond issue for the construction of a County hospital should be approved by the voters of Olmsted County during 1948."[52] Then on September 10, 1948, the county board approved resolutions to hold a referendum with the November 2 general election, "for the erection of a hospital building, including equipment, to be located at the City of Rochester at a cost of not to exceed $750,000."[53]

Dr. Braasch's committee kicked into high gear to gain support for the referendum. It met with twenty-five civic groups in less than two weeks, created posters and sample ballots, and was featured in the *Rochester Post-Bulletin*. They explained that two "yes" votes were required, one to build the hospital and another to issue the bonds to finance it. They also explained that the financing for the new hospital would raise property taxes by only 1.25% over the existing level. Importantly, the Mayo Clinic Board of Governors expressed its support: "The Clinic believes that a hospital built by the community would be of benefit to the health of the residents of Rochester and Olmsted County. It is quite evident that there is a need for more family physicians and general practitioners in this community. We believe that this need can be met only if a Community Hospital with modern facilities is made available to such physicians."[54]

The referendum passed with a 73% majority, 12,496 to 4,564. Rochester-area residents were finally going to have a hospital of their own. Eventually.

---

50 *Rochester Post-Bulletin*, Jan. 9, 1948.
51 *Rochester Post-Bulletin*, Jan. 9, 1948.
52 Olmsted County Board Minutes, Jan. 9, 1948.
53 Olmsted County Board Minutes, Sep. 5, 1948.
54 William F. Braasch papers, Mayo Foundation Historical Section.

Chapter 2
Dr. Wente and the Olmsted Medical Group

In August 1922, Moose Lake, Minnesota, a town of about 800, was still recovering from the huge forest fire that had destroyed that town and thirty-seven others in October 1918, taking 500 lives, Minnesota's worst natural disaster. On August 29, the newborn Harold Alois Wente weighed in at just over twelve pounds on the fish scale in the local hospital, a temporary tar-papered building.[55] Hal, as he became known, was the first child of Aloysious Joseph and Anna Bergfeld Wente who had grown up in German-speaking homes in southern Illinois. A World War I Navy veteran, Hal's father had left his job in Minneapolis two years earlier and struck out for the North Country to make his fortune as a Chevy dealer in Moose Lake. The day after buying the garage, Mr. Wente took a train to Chicago where he proposed to Anna. They married the day after that and took the train back to Moose Lake. Hal's brother Eugene, who became a long-time teacher at Lourdes High School, was born in 1924 and a sister, Maxine, followed in 1925.

The Wentes were one of only two Catholic families and two Democrat families in Moose Lake. Their religious and political leanings were noticed by the local Ku Klux Klan, which burned a cross in their front yard one Saturday night. It didn't seem to have hurt the garage business, though, as a few days after the cross burning, Hal's father found a Klan robe in the back seat of a customer's car. The customer returned to find the indomitable Mr. Wente wearing it. But times changed, and in the 1930s, Al Wente was elected mayor and became involved in statewide politics.

Hal's upbringing was typical of small-town northern Minnesota of the times. When he was old enough, he took on a paper route and then later worked at Ecklund's grocery. Hal also helped at his father's garage, of course. While in high school, he drove one of his dad's trucks, assisting a WPA crew,[56] and he spent one summer on a state highway crew, both jobs arranged by his father, the mayor. Shortly before graduating, Hal announced that he wanted to become a doctor, and his father arranged a summer job for him as an orderly

---

[55] This chapter is taken almost entirely from Dr. Wente's memoirs.
[56] The Works Progress Administration was a depression-era federal program to provide jobs and improve roads, parks, public buildings, etc.

at the newly opened State Hospital for the Insane in Moose Lake, which he had been instrumental in getting built.

In the summer of 1941, the year after the draft started, Hal and Gene decided to enlist in the Navy. Gene was accepted and went into the V-12 program.[57] Hal was rejected because his eyesight wasn't up to the Navy's standards. Having had one year of pre-medical education at the College of St. Thomas, Hal was then commissioned a Second Lieutenant in the Army Reserve, which required him to be in college twelve months a year. He started medical school at the University of Minnesota in March 1943 and received his St. Thomas degree the following spring. During the Hal's first quarter of medical school, the Army announced that medical students could resign their commissions and enlist as privates. They could then take an examination for Army Specialized Training, and if they passed, the Army would pay the remainder of their medical school expenses. If they failed, it was off to war. Hal and most of his class took a chance on the exam, and all passed.

In June 1943, after Mass at the Newman Center at the University of Minnesota, Hal met Elaine Daly of Rochester. They started dating and, after Elaine graduated in March 1944, she decided to stay in Minneapolis near Hal and work as a dental hygienist rather than join the WAF[58] with a friend as she had originally planned. Hal and Elaine were married on June 16, 1945, the day after he finished his junior year of medical school. Their first daughter, Anne, arrived on June 5, 1946, just in time for a move to Milwaukee for a year's internship. After his internship, Dr. Wente reported to Fort Sam Houston in San Antonio for training. From there, he was assigned to Fort Mason in San Francisco for duty as a transport surgeon. He served on Army troopships and hospital ships returning soldiers from the Far East, mostly Japan and the Philippines, making eight voyages. Meanwhile, his brother in the Navy had spent the entire war on shore duty!

After Dr. Wente completed his two years of active duty with the Army at the end of May, 1949, he and Mrs. Wente returned to the Midwest to look for a place to live and work. They stopped in Rochester to leave their two daughters—Mary had been born on April 1, 1948—with her parents while they went looking. One evening in June, Hal met with two former medical

---

[57] An accelerated college and naval officer training program.
[58] Women in the Air Force.

school roommates who were then residents at the Mayo Clinic at the Old Heidelberg Bar, owned by Elaine's uncle and godfather, Joe Daly. They encouraged him not to do a residency, but to stay in Rochester and set up his own general practice. They told him of the plans for a new community hospital and about the referendum that had passed the previous November. This came as exciting news. The Wentes had wanted to live in a small city similar to Rochester but had not considered Rochester itself because of the lack of a hospital Hal could use. Elaine's father suggested that Hal visit with Harry Harwick, the administrator of the Mayo Clinic, to discuss the opportunity.

When Mr. Harwick learned the nature of Dr. Wente's visit, he called in Slade Shuster, who was soon to be his successor. The visit convinced Dr. Wente that Rochester was a great practice opportunity. Mr. Harwick said the Mayo Clinic administration had encouraged Dr. Braasch in his efforts to establish a community hospital, because they believed that another hospital with well-trained physicians would be an asset for the community and good for the Mayo Clinic. Mr. Harwick thought that the local people would appreciate the Mayo Clinic more when they had a choice for their medical care. He said the local hospital would have to be a good hospital because the Mayo Clinic should not and would not tolerate poor medicine in its backyard. "Looking back," Dr. Wente recalled, "I realize this man's vision was the deciding factor in my decision to start a practice in Rochester." Mr. Schuster had also been very friendly that day and continued to be helpful for many years.

The day after his visit with Mr. Harwick, Dr. Wente learned that Dr. Ted Wellner, then Rochester's only full-time general practitioner, was moving his practice from the Lawler Dry Cleaners building to the new First National Bank building. Dr. Wente made a courtesy call but met with a less-than-friendly reception. Dr. Wellner said he didn't think the hospital would ever be built, and he had negative comments about the office he was leaving. Later, he told Dr. Wente that he would have never left the office if he knew that Wente would be renting it. He wasn't particularly interested in having more competition.

The Lawler building, owned by Bill Lawler, a relative of Elaine (all the Rochester Irish were relatives of Elaine), was a two-story brick structure on the southwest corner of Broadway and Center Street. The site is now part of the Center Street parking ramp adjacent to Michael's Restaurant.

Lawler Cleaners was on the first floor, and the second floor was shared by Dr. Wente, an insurance agency, and the auto license bureau. Dr. Wellner had been right about the office; it was the bare minimum needed. It had a 6-by-12-foot lobby, two 12-by-12-foot exam rooms, and a small darkroom for developing X-rays. Dr. Wente purchased equipment from C.F. Anderson Co. of Minneapolis on credit, up to $3,000 at 6%, which was high for the times. He ordered $1,019 worth of furniture and equipment, and an X-ray machine and accessories for $1,800. In only about an hour, the salesman taught him how to take X-rays and develop them. When he wrote up the order, the salesman noted that Dr. Wente had not requested an ear syringe or emesis basin. Dr. Wente had never washed out ears and didn't expect to be doing so. The salesman said he would give Dr. Wente the syringe and basin if he would charge $2 for each ear irrigation and keep a log for one year. If, after one year, Dr. Wente hadn't earned $100, the salesman would buy Dr. Wente dinner at the city's finest restaurant. That first year, Dr. Wente logged $126; he could afford to buy his own dinner.

* * *

Dr. Wente opened his practice on July 15, 1949, as a solo general practitioner with no inkling of what he was starting. Elaine came in a few hours each day as receptionist. Many of her relatives came to see the office that first day, and there were floral arrangements from relatives, pharmacies, the Mayo Clinic, and the creditors. It was quite a party. There were two patients the first day, a man for a prescription renewal and a woman with a cold. Not a particularly auspicious start, but both patients paid cash, $4 total.

Start-up expenses for the new practice included a state medical license and a federal narcotics registration at $1 each, dues for the county and state medical societies and for the American Medical Association, totaling $32 a year, and dues for the Jaycees at $10. Malpractice insurance was $25 for the standard $25,000 in coverage. Office expenses were $509.84 the first month, including rent of $96. Gross income averaged about $1,000 per month through the end of 1949. In August, Dr. Wente hired his first assistant, Mildred Pecinovsky, who came from a farm near Protovin, Iowa. She was a high school graduate with no office skills, but she was remarkably resourceful and energetic, and the patients loved her. She called patients by their first names on the initial visits, which irritated Dr. Wente, but she was so gregarious that it seemed to work. He taught her to take X-rays, to do simple lab tests, and to assist with suturing lacerations and with dressing changes.[59] By the end of 1949, he was seeing about twenty patients a day, thirteen in the office and seven on house calls. These were long days, and Dr. Wente worked seven days a week. The office was open all day Saturday, and he made house calls on Sunday.

By 1951, the practice was really taking off. Dr. Wente saw thirty patients a day, twenty-two in the office and eight on house calls. Gross income had climbed to $2,000 a month, allowing some debt repayment. Dr. Wente saw mostly patients with acute illnesses and accident cases. He cared for minor fractures, but he didn't do office surgery. Both Dr. George L. Joyce and Dr. Ted Wellner, Rochester's other general practitioners, did tonsillectomies and circumcisions in their homes, with their wives giving open-drop ether anesthesia. Dr. Wente was never tempted to try this. He did do spinal taps, which were required by the state for patients with positive blood tests for syphilis. The state laboratory also sent containers for Dr. Wente to collect and submit tuberculosis sputum samples, diphtheria throat cultures, and gonorrhea smears. Another common procedure was peritoneocentesis— withdrawing fluid from the abdominal cavity to diagnose or relieve pressure from cancer or cirrhosis. Insurance and pre-employment exams were an easy source of cash for Dr. Wente and, more importantly, often led to long-term patients. Another source of income, and problems, was examining drunk drivers for the police. The disadvantage was that the drivers were sometimes friends, patients, or other doctors, but Dr. Wente developed a valuable relationship with the law enforcement fraternity.

It quickly became apparent that the greatest medical need in Rochester was for home visits, and as a result Dr. Wente was soon making ten house calls a day, traveling to the ends of the county and beyond, from Pine Island to Stewartville and from Kasson to Eyota. Many patients were "on the county," which only paid 60% of regular charges, but did pay full mileage and, importantly, the county always paid. Dr. Wente recalls house calls as perhaps his greatest medical experiences. While regretting that modern physicians miss these experiences, he wouldn't go back to those days when his two bags carried a limited armamentarium.

---

[59] She stayed about three or four years. Dr. Wente saw her on May 1, 2008, for the first time in years, said she looks great, and lives in Stewartville, Minnesota.

Polio was an annual summertime scourge. In 1952, a particularly bad year for the disease, Dr. Wente got a call about a child having trouble breathing. He put the boy in his car and raced to St. Marys Hospital. Emergency departments were not staffed then as they are today, and only a nun was present. He told the nun to call a surgeon, but the nun replied that there was no time and handed Dr. Wente a scalpel. He gulped hard and started to make his first tracheostomy. Fortunately, a good friend and surgery resident happened by and helped complete the procedure, saving the boy's life.

Many house calls were for other contagious diseases. Measles, mumps, chicken pox, whooping cough, scarlet fever, and rheumatic fever were also rampant at the time, unlike today when immunizations make most of these diseases rarities.

In June 1952, Dr. James Doyle, a friend and former St. Thomas classmate of Dr. Wente, stopped in Rochester to visit a mutual friend from St. Thomas, Dr. Tony Bianco, then a resident at the Mayo Clinic and later a well-known pediatric orthopedic surgeon there. Dr. Doyle had been a chemistry major, not a pre-medical student, so he was not eligible for the Army medical program. Instead, he had enlisted the Army after his second year of college and fought across Europe with the 87th Infantry Division, earning a Silver Star, Bronze Star, and Purple Heart, among other honors. He returned to graduate from the University of Minnesota Medical School in 1949, then served three more years as an Army surgeon in Europe. Dr. Doyle was out of the Army now, waiting to start a pathology residency in six months, and looking for a place to work temporarily. Dr. Bianco told him that Dr. Wente was getting busy and could probably use some help. Dr. Doyle and his wife Mary then visited Dr. Wente in his office, where Dr. Wente gave them a tour and told them of the plans for the new hospital. He also informed the couple that he was looking for a site to build a clinic. The doctors signed a contract and began a long, happy association.[60]

With two doctors working in the tiny office in the Lawler building, it was terribly overcrowded. They tried to have only one doctor in the office at a time, while the other was off duty or making house calls. They also had a unique record system using 5-by-8-inch note cards for both medical and financial information. This was a common practice then, but they added a

[60] Doyle, J.R., Interview, July 17, 1997; Wente memoirs.

colorful twist. Dr. Wente used blue ink and Dr. Doyle green. The after-hours call system consisted of a private phone line with an emergency number in Dr. Wente's house and an extension in Dr. Doyle's. Whoever was off call would simply disconnect the phone.

When it appeared that the new hospital would be built next to the Public Health Center on Fourth Street Southeast, Dr. Wente attempted to buy land for his planned clinic near that site, where Roscoe's Root Beer & Ribs now stands. Unsuccessful in this, he looked at dozens of other sites before settling on a parcel on Third Avenue Southeast. Because of the devastating flood of July 21, 1951, the worst to hit the city since 1908, the county decided not to build the hospital at that Fourth Street location, picturesquely known from its early history as the Buffalo Wallow. (How does Buffalo Wallow Medical Center sound?) Drs. Wente and Doyle were disappointed, but they decided to stay with the Third Avenue property. The property consisted of five lots, three on Third Avenue Southeast and two on 9½ Street Southeast. The land was part of the estate of Dr. Christopher Graham, the second partner of the Mayo brothers and Dr. Charles Mayo's brother-in-law, who had died in July 1952. An 18-room deserted house, a former Van Dusen mansion[61], stood in the middle of this property. Before buying it, Dr. Wente again sought advice from Harry Harwick, who reassured him that it was a good location and that he should purchase all the land he could. Drs. Wente and Doyle planned to build on the lots facing Third Avenue and convert the Van Dusen mansion into apartments. The price for the property was $20,000. The estate also owned twenty acres to the north of the lots Drs. Wente and Doyle were considering, including the mansion in which Mrs. Graham still lived. She was more than 90 years old, and her son-in-law, George Lowrey, who administered the estate, said that that land would also be available when she passed away.

Dr. Wente talked to a local builder, Clarence C. Pagenhart, who had been the leading commercial contractor in Rochester for some years, had done most

---

[61] This was owned by George Washington Van Dusen (1826-1915) from 1905 until his death but was occupied by his son Frank R. Van Dusen. It was sold by G.W.'s estate to Dr. Christopher Graham. G.W. VanDusen, who came to Rochester in 1864, was a successful grain dealer, Rochester's first millionaire, and mayor in 1872 and 1873. He owned elevators and mills all along the Chicago and Northwestern Railway and named the town of Byron after his hometown Port Byron, New York. He moved to Minneapolis in 1890, but is interred in Oakwood Cemetery's largest mausoleum. His son, Frederick, married Dr. Edwin C. Cross's daughter, Myra, in 1884.

of the recent work for the Mayo Clinic and St. Marys, and had built Folwell School. A new firm, Stocke and Company, had recently displaced him in his work for the Mayo Clinic, and he had a personal interest in helping Dr. Wente's new group. Mr. Pagenhart arranged for local architect Daniel Robbins to draw up plans and for the Rochester State Bank to finance the building if Drs. Wente and Doyle could buy the land. The doctors were able to scrape up $5,000 apiece and their attorney Dick Plunkett, later president of the bank, and his brother, Warren, who became a district judge, contributed the other $10,000, and a new enterprise named Medical Properties was formed. Pagenhart insisted that the old mansion be demolished and that the new building be first-class, with brick and stone, air-conditioning, and hot-water heat.

A local artist, Ruth Larson, agreed to take down the old mansion in exchange for the materials, which she wanted to use in the construction of her new home. She and a helper took the mansion apart stone by stone. It turned out that the "stones" were actually 20-by-12-by-12-inch concrete blocks, and it took three or four months to complete the demolition. Drs. Wente and Doyle and the architect worked on the plans for the new building for several months, too. The architect had never designed a medical clinic, and there were no standard plans available. A small clinic of this type was still a rarity; doctors typically rented space in office buildings. The Olmsted Medical Group followed Mayo Clinic's concept of combination consulting, examination, and treatment rooms instead of the usual three separate rooms. Drs. Wente and Doyle added other ideas of their own to complete the plan. Construction began in February, 1953.[62]

The next issue was what to call the clinic. They toyed with several names, but thought they should avoid using "Rochester" or "Clinic" in the name to avoid confusion with the better known clinic in Rochester. Dr. Wente thought it might be diplomatic to discuss the issue with Slade Schuster, who was now the administrator at Mayo Clinic. Mr. Schuster agreed with their concerns and suggested using "Zumbro" in the name. Dr. Wente had considered "Dubuque" because Third Avenue Southeast had been part of the old Dubuque Trail. Mr. Schuster also suggested that they call themselves a group rather than clinic, which appealed to both the partners. They thought that "Olmsted," after the county, sounded better than either "Dubuque" or "Zumbro." Thus, the name "Olmsted Medical Group" came to be.

---

[62] *Rochester Post-Bulletin*, Aug. 21, 1953, p. 10.

By this time, Drs. Wente and Doyle had added a third partner, Dr. John Stransky, a medical school friend of Dr. Wente. Dr. Stransky was an Air Force flight surgeon and arrived at the Rochester airport for an interview in style—piloting a B-24 bomber. He had graduated high in his class and had had an internship and a year of surgical training before joining the Air Force. He liked their new office and they liked him, so he was hired.

On August 17, 1953, the doctors moved into their new building. It was a rectangular one-story building of steel and masonry construction with a brick exterior.[63] There was a small waiting area with an administrative office and a supply closet. Down a hallway were six rooms—an X-ray facility, a lab, and four identical rooms for consultation, examination, and treatment. The arrangement of the desk, exam table, and sinks was the same in each room and had been deliberately designed for efficient patient flow and privacy.

The three partners invited many people from the Mayo Clinic to their grand opening reception, and were a bit surprised that they all actually came. They had one special guest that afternoon, Sen. Hubert Humphrey. Dr. Wente had met him some years earlier when he accompanied his father to a meeting of the Minnesota League of Cities. Their attorney, Dick Plunkett, was chairman of the Olmsted County Democratic Party and had invited Senator Humphrey. Drs. Wente and Doyle were thrilled at the surprise. Dr. Stransky, a staunch Republican, was less so. The *Rochester Post-Bulletin* covered the opening of the Olmsted Medical Group, and the story was picked up by the United Press and appeared in newspapers throughout the country. The new clinic in a built-for-doctors building attracted a lot of interest, and doctors traveled from all over the Midwest to see it.

Although Drs. Wente, Doyle, and Stransky didn't realize it at the time, this was the start of the Olmsted Medical Group as a permanent institution. Typical medical practices were located in rented offices and stayed in business only as long as the doctor practiced. Medical records were then transferred to the patients' new physicians. Only the major clinics like Mayo, Cleveland, and Ochsner had any permanence. Now, the Olmsted Medical Group had a name, a place, and the potential for permanence.

---

[63] The bricklayer was Richard Blondell, who later built and operated the Blondell Motel.

Chapter 3
A Community Hospital at Last

Dr. Wente established his practice in Rochester with the assurance that a community hospital would soon be built. But getting the hospital built turned out to be much harder than passing the 1948 referendum, although the project started out auspiciously enough. On November 8, 1948, the Olmsted County Board of Commissioners held its first meeting after the referendum, made note of the vote and authorized notice of a bond sale, with bids to be opened on December 8. Bids were received from fourteen financial syndicates comprising 43 banks and bond dealers. Only ten days earlier, Moody's had given Olmsted County a AAA rating, its highest and the first ever for a Minnesota bond issue. A syndicate composed of Otis & Co. of Cleveland and the Chicago firms Central Republic Co., Dempsey & Co., and Ballman and Main submitted the winning bid. Mr. Evenson, the bond consultant, said he had never seen such a successful bond offering, a real tribute to Olmsted County.[64, 65, 66]

At its meeting on January 11, 1949, the county board directed the county treasurer to invest $700,000 of the hospital fund in U.S. Treasury notes pending the construction of the hospital. Dr. Braasch, Dr. Viktor Wilson, the county health officer, and Mr. Fred Palen, another member of the Citizens' Voluntary Hospital Committee, appeared before the board to discuss the matter of appointing a county hospital advisory committee. The board then appointed Avery Tews, A.J. Lobb, James O'Connor, and Paul Grassle, with Dr. Braasch as chairman and Dr. Wilson as an ex-officio member.[67]

The first issue for the advisory committee was finding a suitable site for the hospital. They wanted a central location for the convenience of patients, physicians, and Mayo Clinic consultants, but several centrally located properties were too expensive. The committee also wanted the hospital to be close to the Public Health Center, which was already being built on the west side of Bear Creek. Adequate space for parking was important as

---

[64] The AAA rating and resultant low interest rate testified to the county's fiscal responsibility and reliability.
[65] Olmsted County Board Minutes.
[66] *Rochester Post-Bulletin*, Dec. 9, 1948, p. 11.
[67] Olmsted County Board Minutes.

was room for future expansion. Other considerations included noise, smoke, dust, traffic, landscaping, and availability of heat from the city steam plant.[68] The committee recommended considering city-owned land north of Fourth Street Southeast between Bear Creek and Sixth Avenue, across the creek from the health center. This area had been flooded earlier in the year, but the health center had stayed dry and the committee planned to have the hospital elevated an extra two feet. On August 8, 1949, the county board voted to take up the question of the land's availability with the Rochester City Council. On September 9, Ellerbe & Co. was selected as architects for planning the new county hospital. It was already becoming apparent that due to inflation $750,000 was not going to provide the hoped-for hospital. And the smaller hospital they could afford would soon need to be expanded.

The second issue for the committee to tackle was financing, including the question of securing federal Hill-Burton funds which could pay up to 45% of the cost of the project. After investigating the likelihood of obtaining the federal funds, the county board voted to apply, thinking the project could likely be funded within a year.[69] Unfortunately, even though lobbying the Minnesota Department of Health raised the hospital's priority from seventy-second to sixty-fourth of proposed projects for Hill-Burton funds, funding for the program was decreased, and eventually it became obvious that the county was on its own—it had missed the chance for federal funding.[70]

In January 1950, the county board authorized Ellerbe to make tests and soundings for footings for the hospital. In July, Dr. Braasch and Mr. Tews met with the county board to further discuss the site, and the board again decided to meet with the city council about obtaining the property. By the following April, two and a half years after the referendum, there was still no visible progress, and on April 10, Dr. Wente submitted a letter to the board "from the various physicians and surgeons of the county urging action in the erection of the proposed county hospital." Members of the fair board were next on the county board agenda, to discuss new buildings on the fairgrounds.[71] Just five weeks later, the contract was awarded for construction of the new cattle barn.[72] The proposed hospital was clearly not

---

[68] William F. Braasch papers, Mayo Foundation Historical Section.
[69] Olmsted County Board Minutes, Dec. 8, 1949.
[70] William F. Braasch papers, Mayo Foundation Historical Section.
[71] Olmsted County Board Minutes, Apr. 10, 1951.
[72] Olmsted County Board Minutes, May 18, 1951.

the board's first priority. On May 10, the county board appointed Dr. J.S. Lundy, a Mayo Clinic anesthesiologist, to replace Mr. Lobb on the hospital advisory committee. There were now two Mayo Clinic doctors on the committee—but none of the physicians who would actually use the new community hospital.

In June 1951, the board approved the Bear Creek site, the Buffalo Wallow, for the hospital. Dr. Braasch, Dr. Wente, and Mr. E.W. Buenger, Ellerbe's local architect, met with the board on July 10, presented site plans, and asked that the city be requested to transfer the land to the county. The county auditor was instructed to write to the city council that the county desired to acquire the land in question. The hospital advisory committee also asked the county board to establish a temporary laboratory in the Public Health Center, and the board authorized the committee to investigate further the costs and the availability of a laboratory technician.

But in just one day, all that planning was washed away. On Saturday, July 21, 1951, the worst flood since the Great Flood of 1908 swept through Rochester, inundating the proposed hospital site. Despite the studies of past floods and the plan for raising the hospital's elevation, the flood alarmed many people. Petitions were circulated throughout the county and presented to the county board in early 1952 requesting that the hospital not be located at the Buffalo Wallow.[73] The hospital advisory committee looked for alternate sites, even the possibility of remodeling an existing structure, but it ultimately came back to its original recommendation. In a letter to the county board, Dr. Braasch urged that there be no further delay of the project. "The need of the hospital is evident to everyone. The physicians now engaged in general practice are handicapped by the lack of hospital facilities available to them."[74] The possibility then arose of acquiring an irregularly shaped eight-and-a-half-acre parcel of land on the edge of the state hospital property. State hospital, state government, and county officials met at the state hospital to discuss this possibility. Dr. Magnus Petersen, the state hospital superintendent, was supportive, as were other state officials. The State Legislature, in its 1953 session, passed special legislation to allow the state to sell the land to the county for $2,500.[75,76]

---

[73] Olmsted County Board Minutes, Feb. 7, 1952.
[74] William F. Braasch papers, Mayo Foundation Historical Section.
[75] William F. Braasch papers, Mayo Foundation Historical Section.
[76] *Rochester Post-Bulletin*, Sep. 3, 1953, p. 1.

33

With a site selected, it was finally time to begin serious planning for the new community hospital. Dr. Braasch and Mr. Buenger visited more than a dozen small hospitals, collecting ideas and learning about their problems. They also consulted with several medical experts at the Mayo Clinic—but not with any of the future medical staff. The cost estimate for the first plan was more than a third over budget and the hospital had to be pared down. The hospital was reduced from one hundred to fifty-five beds and a number of other components were deleted from the plan. There would be no basement, service or patient elevator, no postoperative recovery room, and no bath or toilet facilities in most rooms. Mr. Buenger presented preliminary plans for the hospital to the county board on March 11, 1953. On June 8, Dr. Braasch, Mr. Buenger, and Paul Grassle reported that the advisory committee and the Minnesota Board of Health had reviewed the plans and were in agreement with them. The county board then accepted the plans and instructed Ellerbe to proceed with final drawings and specifications in preparation for requesting bids for construction. At last, on March 11, 1954, bids were opened, and contracts were awarded the next day: A.O. Stocke Co., $339,670 for general construction; Foster Electric Co., $37,984; and Grudem Brothers, $146,750 for mechanical systems. Equipment bids over the next few months would total almost $96,000.

On April 13, 1954, five and a half years after passage of the referendum, Dr. Braasch and County Board Chairman O.P. Giese finally broke ground for what was now being called the Olmsted Community Hospital—"county hospital" had negative connotations because the term usually denoted a charity institution. Two months later, the hospital's board of directors was appointed. Members were Dr. Braasch, chairman; Mrs. Irene Cysewski, director of nursing at the state hospital; Robert Skar, Jr., a printer; Wendell Lenton, mayor of Stewartville; Harry Evans, a local businessman; M.E. Commigore, a banker in Dover; and John deJ. Pemberton, Jr., an attorney whose father was a Mayo Clinic physician and whose nephew, John deJ. Pemberton III, would be as well.[77]

The hospital board was then authorized to hire an administrator.[78] Dr. Braasch, in his travels among the smaller hospitals in the area, had been

---

[77] Mr. Pemberton did legal work for Mayo and St. Marys. His junior partner, Ron Seeger, later founded Rochester's largest law firm.

[78] Olmsted County Board Minutes, June 15, 1954.

impressed by Cedric Linville, the hospital administrator at Glencoe, Minnesota. A furniture dealer who became active in the campaign to construct that town's hospital, Mr. Linville had become its administrator in 1947. By 1954, its bonds had been paid off and the hospital had cash reserves,[79] a very impressive record in the view of the hospital board. Mr. Linville was appointed administrator of the Olmsted Community Hospital at the salary of $10,000 for the year beginning January 1, 1955.[80]

* * *

Meanwhile, the Olmsted Medical Group had continued to grow, and Dr. Wente was proving that there was more to vision than Navy eye charts. Concerned with the delays in building the hospital, Dr. Stransky worried that his surgical skills would become rusty before it opened, and he left the Olmsted Medical Group after a year to practice in Watertown, South Dakota. His departure meant that Drs. Wente and Doyle had a patient load suitable for three doctors, not two. Dr. Jack Verby, another medical school classmate of Dr. Wente and a friend of Dr. Doyle, had been a star pitcher for the Rochester Queens[81] baseball team and was well known in the area. He had practiced in Litchfield, Minnesota, for two years prior to Army service in Korea. He had returned to Litchfield after his service, but Dr. Wente heard that he was unhappy there and so paid him a visit. Dr. Verby's wife was from Lake City, which helped make Rochester attractive. He started in the summer of 1954, and as an experienced practitioner he contributed much to the Olmsted Medical Group's early success.

The fourth annual scientific meeting of the Minnesota Academy of General Practice was held in Rochester in October 1954. Dr. Wente and Dr. Ray Page of St. Charles were in charge of the program. They met with the Mayo Clinic Board of Governors to secure their cooperation, and the board appointed a committee to work with them. Drs. Page and Wente wanted a series of talks of not more than 20 minutes each on topics that a general practitioner could put to use the next day in the office. Dr. Wente says the Mayo Clinic doctors were shocked. They had never heard of a program like this, with such short time frames, and were concerned that if any speaker talked beyond his time

---

[79] William F. Braasch papers, Mayo Foundation Historical Section.
[80] Olmsted County Board Minutes, Feb. 9, 1955.
[81] Among other names, Rochester, like Cincinnati, has been known as The Queen City.

limit, it would throw the whole program into disarray. In the end, though, they agreed to the format. Eight hundred people registered, and the meeting was a tremendous success. The Mayo Clinic was so impressed that the next April it began a series of annual courses with the same format, eventually called the Mayo Clinical Reviews, a series which continues to this day.[82, 83]

With the "hospital for general practitioners" due to open in June 1955, Dr. Wente believed that it could not succeed unless it had a surgeon and an obstetrician. Dr. John Watson, who had just completed a Mayo Clinic residency in obstetrics and gynecology, joined the Olmsted Medical Group in January 1955. He had been in Elaine Wente's class at Rochester High School, and his wife was a friend of Elaine's from college. His father was chairman of the board of the Kahler Corporation, and his brother was president. Dr. Watson began taking on obstetrical patients immediately, and when the hospital opened in June, he had a number of patients ready to deliver babies there. Dr. Mary Price also joined the Olmsted Medical Group in January. A native of Scotland, she had completed an ophthalmology residency at Mayo Clinic. She would be married January 26 to George Pougiales, a local attorney and another high school classmate of Elaine Wente.

Later that winter, the Olmsted Medical Group also hired its first fully qualified residency-trained surgeon, Dr. Harry Burich, who was to start July 1. A native of Silver Lake, Minnesota, Dr. Burich graduated from the University of Minnesota and completed a surgical residency at the university. He then worked for two years at the Gundersen Clinic in La Crosse. As more surgeons named Gundersen joined the staff, he felt that his future advancement there might be limited. In medical school, Dr. Burich had been a friend of Dr. Verby, who informed him of the opportunity in Rochester.[84] Dr. Burich went on to become the backbone of the surgery department for 27 years. The Olmsted Medical Group now had three specialists as well as three general practitioners. With the practice doing so well, the Olmsted Medical Group made the first of four additions to its building, including six more patient rooms and enlarged waiting and administrative areas.

---

[82] Wente memoirs.

[83] Programs in Wente papers, Olmsted Medical Center Archive.

[84] Burich, H.F., Interview, May 25, 2007.

When Orville Freeman became governor of Minnesota in January 1955, he appointed Dr. Wente to the Minnesota State Board of Health. On April 12 that year, the Food and Drug Administration announced the success and licensing of the Salk polio vaccine. The state board of health quickly approved its use in Minnesota for pregnant women, and soon thereafter for the state's general population. The Olmsted Medical Group was the first facility in Rochester and one of the first in the state to offer the vaccine. Shot clinics were held in the evenings after regular office hours. People lined up around the block, eager to avoid the devastating disease, an annual summertime terror. These shot clinics gave many future patients their first and favorable introduction to the Olmsted Medical Group and its office. They were also an indicator of the high quality of modern medical care that Dr. Wente and the Olmsted Medical Group were prepared to deliver to the community.

* * *

The Olmsted Community Hospital medical staff was organized on January 21, 1955. Charter members were Drs. Doyle, Price, Verby, Watson, and Wente from the Olmsted Medical Group; Drs. Joyce and Wellner from Rochester; Dr. H.M. Skaug, Chatfield; Dr. E.W. Ellis, Elgin; Drs. C.B. McKaig and E.A. Olson, Pine Island; Drs. R.A. Glabe and D.G. Mahle, Plainview; Drs. R.L. Page and Pat Rollins, St. Charles; and Dr. Al Risser, Stewartville. Dr. D.E. Affeldt from Kasson was added to the charter list on February 25 because his application had been mislaid. Dr. Burich and Drs. C.G. Ochsner and L.M. Eckstrand from Wabasha also were added to the staff that evening, but not as charter members.[85]

Having specialists such as Drs. Watson and Burich in the "general practitioners' hospital" was not exactly what Dr. Braasch and most of the other community leaders had in mind. Dr. Braasch publicly announced that this was a hospital for general practitioners only and that no specialists should be allowed on the active staff. It appeared to Dr. Wente that Dr. Braasch felt that the Olmsted Medical Group had overstepped its bounds. Dr. Wente recalled that at that February 1955 medical staff meeting, Dr. Braasch, tall and dignified at 76, pointed a "long bony finger" at him and declared, "Dr. Wente, you are not going to control this hospital."[86] Because of this, when

---

[85] Olmsted Community Hospital Medical Staff Minutes.
[86] Wente memoirs. Consistent with Olmsted Community Hospital Medical Staff Minutes, Feb. 25, 1955.

asked to be the first chief of staff of the hospital, Dr. Wente declined and instead suggested Dr. Wellner, who was happy to accept. Dr. Wente never wanted the job anyway, and so he had a good excuse never to take it.[87, 88]

At the same staff meeting, Drs. Wente and McKaig were appointed to plan for a blood supply and ambulance service. The Mayo Clinic blood bank required replacement of two units for each unit used, so the Olmsted Community Hospital reached an agreement with the War Memorial Blood Bank in St. Paul. But blood bank services would be a continuing issue for years.

The new hospital needed an ambulance service to transport acutely ill patients to it. There were two existing ambulance services in Rochester, which belonged to Mayo Clinic and the city. The Mayo Clinic had two converted hearses staffed by general service employees with minimal first aid training. When needed at night, the drivers would have to be called from home for the ambulance run. The city had an old Packard ambulance that was parked in a garage near the police station and was used by the police if the Mayo Clinic service was not available. Dr. Wente approached the police chief (another of Elaine's relatives) about upgrading that service. He was informed that the city council had already refused funds or personnel for that purpose. He then approached Mr. Schuster, the Mayo Clinic administrator, to ask if the Mayo Clinic ambulance service could also serve the Olmsted Community Hospital, but he was turned down. In fact, Mr. Schuster told him the Mayo Clinic had been trying unsuccessfully to sell the ambulance service to a Twin Cities firm, which didn't believe it could be profitable.

Undaunted, Dr. Wente hatched a scheme. He didn't think an Olmsted Medical Group or Olmsted Community Hospital ambulance service would be successful, so instead the Olmsted Medical Group donated the cost of a Ford station wagon ambulance to the local Teamsters union. The Teamsters then purchased the ambulance and donated it to a new service operated by Glenn Bundy and Russ Ruegg, the young owners of the gas station Dr. Wente used, located across from St. Marys where the Blondell Motel now stands. Glenn and Russ took a first aid course and were in business the week before the Olmsted Community Hospital opened. Hardly any patients paid their ambulance bills so it was not a financial success, but the two

[87] Wente memoirs.
[88] Olmsted Community Hospital Medical Staff Minutes, Feb. 25, 1955.

men had minimal overhead and they liked the excitement of the runs. The establishment of a first-class, modern ambulance service in 1962 by Gold Cross spelled the end of the ambulance runs for the gas station owners, and they gave the station wagon back to the Teamsters. Gold Cross went on to acquire the Mayo Clinic ambulance service in 1964, and 30 years later, things came full circle when the Mayo Clinic acquired Gold Cross in 1994.

* * *

The new hospital was completed with the usual change orders, with irregularities in the bids for the sterilizer requiring rebidding, and with issues with sidewalks and sewer and gas lines. The furniture supplier was crippled by a strike, and a new supplier was found just days before the opening. Miss Julia Marchant (later Mrs. Frederick Bohmbach) was appointed director of nursing. From Winnipeg, she had graduated from nursing school in 1934 and circled the globe twice by 1942, including working two years in India. She had originally come to Rochester to work in obstetrics at St. Marys Hospital. Mrs. David Utz, the wife of a Mayo Clinic urologist and a high school classmate of Elaine Wente, was obstetrics supervisor, and Mrs. Hazel Katz was surgery supervisor. Jim Cannady was one of the original employees, an orderly of whom we will hear more later. Francis "Shorty" Daywittt was employed soon after and served as a custodian for four decades.

The dedication of the Olmsted Community Hospital on Sunday, June 26, 1955, was a grand event. The Stewartville High School band played. Mr. Pemberton of the hospital board was the master of ceremonies. Speakers included Dr. Charles Mayo on "Community Health" and the famous medical columnist and Rochester native Dr. Walter C. Alvarez on "The Role of the General Practitioner." Dr. Braasch spoke, too, as well as Dr. Wellner, County Commissioner Richard Towey, Mr. Linville, and Dr. Charles C. Cooper, director of the American Academy of General Practitioners. The invocation was by Rev. G.P. Sheridan, and the benediction by Monsignor Louis O'Day. After the ceremony, three thousand people toured the new hospital. Silver tea service was provided by the Ladies' Auxiliary, the first hospital auxiliary in Rochester, and still a point of pride more than 50 years later.[89] Two days after the dedication, on Tuesday, June 28, 1955, the Olmsted Community Hospital opened at last.

---

[89] Dedication Program, Olmsted Community Hospital, from Wente papers and Braasch papers.

Chapter 4
Boom Times

When the Olmsted Community Hospital opened in the summer of 1955, Rochester was a slowly growing rural town of 30,000 residents about halfway between Hayfield and Plainview and, oddly enough, with a major medical center. The following year, everything changed. On February 8, 1956, the *Rochester Post-Bulletin* reported that IBM would open a research and manufacturing facility in Rochester that would eventually employ 1,500 people. IBM began operations on August 27 in a temporary facility with 174 employees. The company grew to several times that initial projection, and the city's population grew rapidly along with it, adding about 10,000 people per decade, with even more settling throughout the county and in nearby towns. Many young families came to Rochester, and many of them received their healthcare from the young Olmsted Medical Group and the Olmsted Community Hospital.

Shortly after the hospital opened, Dr. Wente met with Dr. Beryl Kirklin, who was the head of the Mayo Clinic radiology department and was facing mandatory retirement from Mayo Clinic at age 65. Rather than stop practicing, he joined the Olmsted Medical Group, the first of several Mayo Clinic retirees to do so. He served the Olmsted Medical Group until his premature death in March 1957. In the summer of the same year, the Olmsted Community Hospital hired Dr. Cyril Corrigan of St. Paul, a distant cousin of Elaine Wente, to practice radiology at the hospital. He also read films for the Olmsted Medical Group part time, joining full-time in 1972.

By late 1955, Dr. Wente began to think about changing the structure of the growing Olmsted Medical Group partnership to facilitate its growth and development. A new partnership agreement was approved on December 1, which created an executive committee to manage the practice and, among other things, stated explicitly that one purpose of the Olmsted Medical Group was "to afford gratuitous administrations to the distressed and indigent." While the Olmsted Medical Group had always cared for anyone regardless of ability to pay, this explicit statement could be regarded as the first step in its evolution to a nonprofit organization. Dr. Wente also seriously considered the business side of the Olmsted Medical Group. Most of his business education had come from reading *Medical Economics*, a popular business magazine for doctors. In 1956, he decided that the Olmsted

Medical Group would benefit from having a management consultant review its operations. He chose Millard Mills from Waterloo, Iowa, who had written for *Medical Economics*. Dr. Burich agreed, and the other partners reluctantly went along, despite the price of $300 for a three-day visit. Mr. Mills was rather scathing in his review. The office staff, he told them, were unhappy, and the doctors were underproductive and didn't charge enough for their services, which would become a recurring theme. To solve the problems, the doctors decided that it was time to hire an administrator.

Olmsted Medical Group administrators were a rare commodity in 1956. There were few group practices, and most of the administrators were self-taught on the job. Dr. Wente sought advice from a classmate, Dr. George Lund of the newly formed St. Louis Park Clinic, which had recently hired an administrator. The Olmsted Medical Group interviewed two candidates and hired Frank J. Wilkus, age 33, who served in the Marines with Carlson's Raiders during World War II and was wounded at Tarawa in the South Pacific. He graduated from St. Thomas University with a bachelor of business administration degree, studied accounting for two years at the University of Minnesota, and took courses in contract law at the St. Paul School of Law. Mr. Wilkus was working at the time in the Minnesota Department of Taxation. He started with the Olmsted Medical Group on April 15, and within about a year, he had replaced the office manager and the disgruntled employees. Mr. Wilkus began to train the doctors in business, instituting double-entry bookkeeping among other reforms, while Dr. Wente trained him in medical practice. This was a fruitful exchange, and according to Dr. Wente, Frank Wilkus became to the Olmsted Medical Group what Harry Harwick had been to the Mayo Clinic. Mr. Wilkus also became involved in local civic affairs, serving three terms on the Rochester City Council from 1968 to 1974 and serving about 25 years on the city's park board.[90]

Dr. Wente had his own foray into politics in 1956. He had been active at the precinct level of the Democratic Party for some time, but now went national. Adlai Stevenson was campaigning for another shot at President Eisenhower and was opposed by Sen. Kefauver of Tennessee and Minnesota's Senator Humphrey. Dr. Wente supported his friend, Senator Humphrey. Senator Kefauver won the Minnesota primary and Stevenson was renominated. Dr. Wente and Dick and Warren Plunkett decided that Senator Humphrey had a

[90] Wente memoirs; Wilkus, F.J., Interview, Aug. 29, 2007.

good chance for the vice presidential nomination and set off for Chicago with 500 newly minted Stevenson-Humphrey buttons, registering at the Hilton as the Stevenson-Humphrey Committee. They had quite an adventure, but it was Stevenson-Kefauver losing again to President Eisenhower.

The Olmsted Medical Group added six new physicians in 1956. In the summer, another general practitioner, Dr. Joe Teynor, came on board. Shortly afterward, Dr. John Flanary walked into Dr. Wente's office and announced that he was from St. Charles, where his father was a veterinarian. He had graduated from Marquette University Medical School[91] and was planning to practice in Rochester. "Why don't you hire me so I don't have to set up an office?" he asked. Dr. Wente explained that they didn't need another doctor and didn't have the space anyway—the second addition had recently been completed and work had already started on the third. But Dr. Flanary persisted, saying that he would work odd hours when space was available. It was an offer Dr. Wente couldn't resist. Dr. Flanary turned out to be a hard worker and did well in his practice. There was no more land for further additions, so Dr. Wente convinced the partners to open a second office, which he and Dr. Flanary staffed, located above Snyder's Drug Store at the Miracle Mile shopping center. A few months later, a fire destroyed the second floor and the medical office was moved to a first-floor storefront location in the shopping center, next to the Red Owl supermarket, the newest and finest grocery in town at the time. This may have been the very first shopping mall doctors' office.

The first of many resident spouses,[92] Dr. Mary Obert, joined the Olmsted Medical Group on a part-time basis in internal medicine in 1956 while she waited for her husband to finish his residency in pathology the next year. In October, Dr. Malcolm Campbell became the Olmsted Medical Group's first full-time internist and a mainstay of that department until his retirement in 1990. He was a fourth-generation physician, born in Iowa and a graduate of the University of Iowa and its medical school. After further training at the University of Illinois, Boston City Hospital, and Minneapolis General Hospital, he served two years in the Army in Korea. He completed a

---

[91] Now the Medical College of Wisconsin.
[92] Hired for temporary positions, several resident spouses became long-term staff members, and the Olmsted Medical Group was even able to hire two of the residents when their training was finished.

fellowship at the University of Minnesota where he was very highly regarded, but he wasn't interested in academia. After Dr. Watson contacted him, Dr. Campbell talked to some internists he knew at the Mayo Clinic. With their encouragement, he joined the Olmsted Medical Group. He provided the quality medical backup that Drs. Burich and Watson needed, and his strong educational background gave the Olmsted Medical Group more credibility with the Mayo Clinic physicians.[93] At the same time, the Olmsted Medical Group added a second surgeon, Dr. Bill Weyhrauch, who had served in the Army Air Corps in the Pacific before attending Carleton College and the University of Minnesota Medical School. He interned in Chicago before completing his residency back at the University of Minnesota.

Dr. John Brodhun was another important addition to the Olmsted Medical Group in 1956. He was born in 1928 in Cologne, Germany. His father was a German machine tool engineer working in Coventry, England. His mother returned to Cologne to give birth so her child would have German citizenship. On a return visit to Germany in 1934, John's father, a World War I veteran, was outspoken in his criticism of Hitler, and he was advised to get out of the country quickly, while he still could—and they did that very night, driving into Belgium. John lived through the six months' bombing of Coventry, sleeping in the air raid shelter at night and, during the day, collecting bomb and shell fragments, which the boys traded like baseball cards. John came to the United States in the fall of 1941 when his father was transferred to work on war production in America. He grew up in Birmingham, Michigan, and attended the University of Michigan and Marquette University Medical School. Late in his Air Force service, Dr. Brodhun decided he wanted to practice in a small town near Milwaukee and listed his availability in the *Wisconsin Medical Journal*. Mr. Wilkus saw the notice and invited Dr. Brodhun to visit Rochester. Dr. Brodhun decided to join the Olmsted Medical Group and stayed with the Wilkuses while he took the state medical licensing exam and looked for a house to buy. But due to the local economic boom, fueled by IBM, affordable houses were in short supply. After searching unsuccessfully, Dr. Brodhun decided he would have to look for another practice elsewhere, where homes were less expensive. He was planning to leave Rochester on a Sunday afternoon, but that morning, a real estate agent called with a house to show him. Dr. Brodhun bought it and went on to become a key leader of the Olmsted Medical Group.[94]

---

[93] Wente memoirs; Campbell, M.A., Interview, Aug. 10, 2007.
[94] Brodhun, J.A., Interview, Sep. 11, 2007; Wente memoirs; Wilkus interview.

By 1957, as IBM was just becoming established in Rochester, the Olmsted Medical Group had already grown to 11 physicians in two buildings, with a professional administrator. It was just the beginning, and the Olmsted Medical Group partners knew that they had to look beyond just adding more physicians and the office space to accommodate them. For one thing, the partners felt that their patients were inconvenienced by the lack of a nearby pharmacy. So in October 1956, they leased a small parcel of land on the north side of the office and constructed a small building for a pharmacy. But because a building to house only a pharmacy would be too small to be practical, they also included space for a dental office. Dick Hargesheimer, who owned the Eagle Drug Store downtown, opened the Apothecary Shop in the new building. Dick Rossi, a Rochester native who had been practicing dentistry in Plainview for seven years, was the first dentist to rent the dental office space. His practice was very successful, and after eight years he moved to a new office in Northwest Rochester, an area that was growing rapidly after IBM's arrival. Doug Nelson moved into the dental office for a time, also did well, and then moved to the new Valhalla dental building off Elton Hills Drive.

Dr. Lloyd Wood, a general practitioner who was practicing in White Bear Lake, joined the Olmsted Medical Group in May 1958. Dr. Wente considered him a great addition, someone who was always willing to volunteer when any extra effort was needed and very popular with patients. In 1963, Dr. Wood left to enter a residency in physical medicine and rehabilitation at the Mayo Clinic. While he stayed on staff at Mayo Clinic, he continued to be a good friend of the Olmsted Medical Group. In July 1958, Mary Doyle's brother, Dr. John Fluegel, joined the Olmsted Medical Group in the Miracle Mile office with Dr. Wente, replacing Dr. Flanary, who had left for an obstetrics residency.[95] Dr. Fluegel stayed only until early 1966 when he left for a psychiatry residency at the University of Minnesota.

* * *

Meanwhile, at the Olmsted Community Hospital, the medical staff was dealing with its own important issues. Hospital staff bylaws had to be approved by both the hospital staff and the board and were then binding on

---

[95] Dr. Flanary practiced in Wisconsin, retired to Florida, and died Mar. 25, 2008; he is buried in St. Charles.
Rochester Post-Bulletin, Jun. 14, 2008, p. B2.

both. While the hospital board didn't like that the staff bylaws were binding on them, they eventually agreed, as this was required for accreditation. A dentist, Dr. Matthew Eusterman, and a podiatrist, Dr. Robert Sabbann, applied for staff privileges at the hospital, but there was no provision for those professions in the bylaws. The staff created a subsidiary dental consulting staff but saw no need for a "chiropodist." Eventually, in 1962, the Joint Commission for Accreditation of Hospitals clarified the issues related to podiatry, the hospital changed its rules, and Dr. Sabbann practiced at the hospital until his retirement in 1994.

Dr. Wente, eager to help the new hospital be successful and always the forward thinker, proposed a package rate for tonsillectomies, combining doctor and hospital charges in a flat fee. His idea was too radical at the time, but it became a prominent part of the 2008 Minnesota state health reform legislation as "baskets of care."

There were early problems with hospital staffing levels, which slowed lab and nursing services, and there were ongoing difficulties obtaining the proper equipment. Mr. Linville seemed agreeable to the doctors' requests for staff and equipment, but was slow to deliver. He reported to the county board, not the doctors, and his primary objective was keeping the hospital financially sound. The doctors would sometimes go to Dr. Braasch to ask him to influence Mr. Linville, but without much success.

Before the December 1955 medical staff meeting, Dr. Louis Buie, the famous Mayo Clinic colon and rectal surgeon, gave a clinical talk, starting an educational practice that has continued to the present in one form or another at the hospital.

The physicians from outside Rochester weren't willing to take emergency department call, and neither was Dr. Joyce, who was from Rochester. Dr. Wellner eventually dropped out, too, leaving only the Olmsted Medical Group physicians to staff it. Use of the Olmsted Community Hospital also declined among the doctors who were not part of the Olmsted Medical Group. At first, some of the physicians from outside Rochester did some surgery at the hospital and delivered babies there. But the location was somewhat inconvenient for them, and they gradually drifted away except for Dr. Al Risser from Stewartville. Dr. Risser was tall and thin, a gentleman in the true sense—nearly saintly. He led a pietist religious group and was very calm, quiet, and soft-spoken. He and his patients were mutually devoted. He delivered babies for many years, and performed minor operations and assisted on major ones almost until his retirement in 1994.

The withdrawal of physicians from outside Rochester did not affect the success of the Olmsted Community Hospital, though. It quickly became popular because of its family-like atmosphere and its smaller, friendlier, more personal scale. Like many families, the hospital even had a garden, one about fifty feet square that was started by the cook, Miss Pearl Granger, and tended by custodian Duane "Dewey" Melvin when he had time. It boasted the usual vegetables as well as rhubarb and even grapevines. There was also a flower garden at the front of the hospital. But as the hospital and Dewey got busier, the gardens could be maintained for only a few years.[96] Rhubarb continued to grow near the hospital, though, until it fell to the 1986 addition.

The downsized hospital was soon inundated with patients. By its first anniversary, there had been 2,334 patients admitted to the hospital, 1,996 outpatient visits, 496 births, and 998 surgical cases.[97] With numbers increasing monthly, the acute shortage of beds was now becoming chronic. On December 27, 1956, just one day less than 18 months after the hospital opened, the medical staff wrote to the county board to request the formation of a committee to study the capacity problem and hospital expansion. Mr. Linville stated in his annual report that "there has been some discussion by the medical staff for building an addition to the hospital. However your administrator cannot see any need at the present time or in the near future." A building advisory committee was appointed anyway, consisting of Calvin T. Slatterly, Henry T. Maass, S.A. Kuhlman, James Jones, and William Friedrich. At the hospital staff meeting in September 1957, it was reported that the committee had met with the county board to discuss a proposed addition that included three operating rooms, two delivery rooms, a second elevator, and more patient rooms. Mr. Linville reported that the hospital was first in line for federal Hill-Burton funds, but plans would need to be completed by July 1958. Drs. Braasch and Verby were opposed to using federal funds for fear of federal controls.[98] In March 1958, the staff was told that the 50-bed addition would cost $556,000 and that Hill-Burton funds

---

[96] Melvin, D., Interview, Apr. 30, 2008.
[97] *Rochester Post-Bulletin*, July 2, 1956.
[98] Olmsted Community Hospital Medical Staff Minutes, Sep. 24, 1957.

would finance $187,000. In June, the county board voted unanimously not to expand the hospital.[99]

The medical staff continued to deal with routine issues, and some that were not so routine. In April 1958, it recommended that the hospital participate[100] with Blue Cross and assist patients with their paper work. In June, the staff wrote to the county board asking that a medical staff member be appointed to the hospital board, but it would be 20 years before that happened. In January 1959, the medical staff endorsed fluoridation of public water supplies. In July, the Olmsted Medical Group took over the entire responsibility for staffing the emergency department due to problems with the emergency call system. In January 1960, the staff donated film to the hospital auxiliary for photographing newborns for their parents. Drs. Wellner and Verby opposed this, thinking it to be unethical promotion.[101] The hospital utilization for 1959 increased to 2,590 inpatients, 3,756 outpatients, 852 births, and 1,394 operations.

The September 1961 medical staff meeting featured a spirited discussion concerning surgical privileging and the appropriate procedures for a general practitioner to perform. Dr. Ellis, the general practitioner from Elgin, pointed out that the hospital was originally for general practitioners and said he was concerned that their privileges could be restricted. Dr. Fluegel, also a general practitioner, stated, "The quickest way for general practitioners to lose their privileges would be for some unfortunate incident to occur and general practitioner surgery would be limited by people not coming to the hospital. We need to keep standards on the highest plane." Dr. Burich said that anyone doing surgery should have surgical training. The staff voted to have the credentials and by-laws committee make future decisions on individual physicians based on their training and experience. At the March 1962 meeting, the staff adopted a recommended policy that it was not safe to give general anesthesia to patients who were not in the hospital the night before. This practice persisted until 1976, when Dr. Burich recommended repealing the hospital rule requiring admission the day before surgery, and the staff agreed.[102] This latter action presaged many additional efforts to

---

[99] Olmsted County Board Minutes, June 10, 1958.

[100] Meaning to accept Blue Cross' payment rates and to be paid directly by the health plan.

[101] This was before doctors and hospitals were allowed to advertise.

[102] Olmsted Community Hosptial Medical Staff Minutes, Mar. 27, 1975; Dec. 2, 1976.

reduce hospital lengths of stay over the next decades. Also approved at the meeting was a routine nursery order sheet, the first step toward what are now called clinical pathways or protocols, which are standardized treatment plans for common conditions.

By 1961, the number of births in the hospital had risen to 917 and there were 1,010 surgical procedures. Admissions were approaching 3,000, a number then typically seen at a 100-bed hospital, not one of 55 beds. The obstetrics area was especially overcrowded, and patients were being discharged earlier than usual to make room. The twelve-bassinet nursery held as many as twenty-four newborns. On November 28, 1961, Drs. Wente, Fluegel, and Risser, along with Dr. Cleon Holland, a local general practitioner, Dr. James Hunter, an obstetrician in solo practice, and Mr. Linville met informally with the county board to again urge expansion of the hospital by about fifty beds and another delivery room. Dr. Risser also wanted to add swing beds, which function as an intermediate stage between hospital and nursing facilities. Dr. Wente pointed out that federal Hill-Burton funds were now available to cover 55% of the expansion cost.[103] On May 8, 1962, the hospital board attended the county board meeting to urge immediate action on expanding the hospital.[104] After detailed discussions between the two boards and architects from Ellerbe, the cost of the expansion was set at $750,000, with $337,500 available from federal funds and $412,500 to be raised from the sale of revenue certificates and repaid wholly from hospital revenues.

But, as with the 1948 referendum, this agreement was not the same as actually building the hospital addition. In March 1963, the medical staff received a letter from Robert Skaar, the president of the hospital board, informing them that the long-planned expansion of the hospital had been suspended indefinitely. The last of the original $750,000 in bonds were retired in December 1964. The hospital had had positive operating margins each year; it had required no taxpayer support beyond the construction of the building.[105]

* * *

---

[103] *Rochester Post-Bulletin*, Nov. 29, 1961.
[104] Olmsted County Board Minutes, May 8, 1962.
[105] *Rochester Post-Bulletin*, Dec. 15, 1964, p. 17.

The Olmsted Medical Group had also been experiencing growing pains of its own, and conflicts began arising. The first controversy was over who should be partners. Most medical groups at that time—not that there were that many—restricted ownership to the early partners, as had the Mayo Clinic. The founding partners of those groups wanted to maintain control of the group's culture and direction and avoid the possibility of being voted out by newcomers, who could take over the practice the partners had worked so hard to establish. Drs. Wente, Doyle, Verby, Watson, and Burich were the partners, while other doctors were employees. The new physicians started agitating to become partners as well. Dr. Wente, ever the liberal, was agreeable to this, but Dr. Verby was not. Ultimately, the partnership was opened to any physician who was employed for at least one year and was approved by the partners. This was a forward-looking move, very unusual for the time, and a significant factor in the Olmsted Medical Group's success and its evolving philosophy. Partly because of this conflict, though, two more doctors left—Drs. Flanary and Teynor.

Medical Properties, the building partnership, also became the subject of controversy. The non-partners saw profits going to this group and particularly resented having Mr. Plunkett, the Olmsted Medical Group's attorney and not a physician, sharing in the profits, forgetting that there would not have been a Olmsted Medical Group building without him. Each partner in the practice was offered the opportunity to buy in to Medical Properties, but not all could afford to or wanted to. This controversy helped prompt two more doctors to leave the Olmsted Medical Group in 1959—Drs. Watson and Weyhrauch.

By 1960, the Olmsted Medical Group was again outgrowing its facilities, and Medical Properties leased land on the west side of Highway 52, south of 19th Street, and contracted with Ray Arend to construct a 5,000-square-foot building and lease it to the Olmsted Medical Group. They held a contest to name the site, and Elaine Wente suggested the winner, "Hillcrest," by which the area is still known. The new office opened on April 1, 1961, replacing the Miracle Mile office. Drs. Wente, Fluegel, and Wood staffed the new office, and Drs. Pougiales and Doyle worked there part-time. An addition was soon built, with more exam rooms, a dental office, and a Ruffalo pharmacy. The new building and the lease arrangement caused more tension within the Olmsted Medical Group over who was profiting and by how much.

In October 1959, soon after the departure of Dr. Watson, a new obstetrician, Dr. Werner Kaese, joined the Olmsted Medical Group. He was from

Pennsylvania, the son of German immigrants, and had learned English in grade school. He graduated from Albright College and the University of Maryland Medical School. He served two years in the Navy as a physician at the United States Naval Academy in Annapolis, Maryland, and then completed a residency in obstetrics and gynecology at Temple University. He was 31, but to Dr. Wente looked more like fifteen. Dr. Verby hired Dr. Kaese while Dr. Wente was away, and Dr. Wente later confessed to Dr. Kaese that he personally would never have hired him. He went on to become the soul of Olmsted Medical Group's obstetrics department for the next thirty-seven years. Dr. Kaese delivered more babies than anyone else in Rochester, including the children of women who he had previously delivered. His wife, Dottie, was a nurse who worked in the obstetrics department at the Olmsted Community Hospital for a number of years.

Several years after he joined the Olmsted Medical Group, Dr. Kaese attended a conference in New York and heard about a new procedure called laparoscopy. He learned that it was being performed at Chicago's Cook County Hospital, and, intrigued, made a call and was warmly invited to a conference and demonstration there. He discovered that the other attendees were academic department chairs, not community practitioners like he was. The conference hosts had simply assumed that Dr. Kaese from Rochester was from the Mayo Clinic. They made him welcome anyway, and he became the first to perform laparoscopic surgery in Rochester, at the Olmsted Community Hospital.[106]

The Olmsted Medical Group still needed a second surgeon, and Dr. Frank V. Sander joined in October 1961. Dr. Sander had graduated summa cum laude from Princeton, received his medical degree from Columbia University, and had his surgical training in Pennsylvania and Michigan, where he had been practicing. Early in his tenure, he was reprimanded for excessive swearing in the operating room. A legendary incident occurred one day when Dr. Risser was assisting him on an apparently difficult case and Dr. Sander was cursing away. "Maybe, Frank," said Dr. Risser, in his quiet voice, "you should try praying."

The partnership model was becoming increasingly unwieldy, and it became clear that the Olmsted Medical Group needed a change in its organizational

---

[106] Kaese, W.E., Interview, Sep. 7, 2007.

structure. As early as 1956, Dr. Wente had talked about some type of corporate structure for the Olmsted Medical Group. In 1961, the Minnesota State Legislature, in its special session mainly devoted to the taconite tax, passed a law permitting professional groups to incorporate. At the urging of Dr. Wente, Mr. Plunkett, and Mr. Wilkus, the Olmsted Medical Group became one of Minnesota's first professional associations, on December 5, 1961. The first articles of incorporation listed all the partners as directors and created two classes of stock to protect the early partners. However, on December 24, 1962, at the first shareholders meeting, revised articles were adopted that created a five-member board of directors, a single class of shares, and a provision that the Olmsted Medical Group could own or lease real estate. Drs. Wente, Doyle, Verby, Burich, and Campbell were elected as directors. Because the Olmsted Medical Group had fewer than 10 shareholders, it chose to become a Subchapter S corporation, so that the individuals would be taxed on their shares of the profits rather than having the corporation pay the tax. This was still a simple organization, one step beyond a partnership. A profit-sharing retirement plan was established for the doctors and the Olmsted Medical Group employees. Mr. Plunkett was the original trustee, but was succeeded by Drs. Burich and Wente in 1972. The IRS refused to approve the plan because its regulations did not recognize professional corporations or their ability to have retirement plans. Each year, the IRS sent a form to be signed, to waive the statute of limitations, keeping the case against the Olmsted Medical Group open until the IRS eventually lost a series of cases in federal courts and changed its regulations.[107] On May 22, 1970, the IRS finally conceded and sent a letter approving the trust.

Dr. Clayton Bennett joined the Olmsted Medical Group in December 1962. He was from Colorado originally, but his wife was from Rochester and had a large extended family in the area. He picked up many of Dr. Wood's patients and built a large practice. The Bennetts owned a farm in Oronoco Township on the south bank of the Zumbro River. For a number of winters, they held a picnic with a bonfire near the river, where staff burned hot dogs and marshmallows in between sledding, skiing, and snowmobiling. The Olmsted Medical Group staff enjoyed this very much, probably even better than summer picnics.

---

[107] http://www.taxlinks.com:80/rulings/1970/revrul70-101.htm

Another obstetrician, Dr. Charles Field, also joined the Olmsted Medical Group in 1962. He had had a general practice in Cresco, Iowa, for several years, and then completed a residency at Mayo Clinic. He became very popular with both the patients and staff; Dr. Wente described him as a cross between Mark Twain and Will Rogers. Dr. Field's growing practice added to the pressures on the hospital facilities.

At the February 1963 board meeting, Dr. Verby suggested that the Olmsted Medical Group start a physical therapy department. This prompted Dr. Burich and Mr. Wilkus to visit several physical therapy facilities in the area. A space was then created in the northwest corner of the Third Avenue building, and the physical therapy department opened on November 28. Gwen Gunsalus worked half-time as the physical therapist in the department for more than 20 years. Dr. Verby announced in July 1963 that he would be participating in the University of Minnesota Medical School's new medical student preceptorship program, a fateful decision, since it would ultimately result in his departure from the Olmsted Medical Group. That fall, the Olmsted Medical Group's garage, which is still used by maintenance, was built behind the Third Avenue building at a cost of $1,300.[108]

Continuing to expand its specialty services, the Olmsted Medical Group added a pediatrics department in 1964 that was staffed by Dr. Thomas Peyla and Dr. James Hartfield. Dr. Peyla had visited Rochester in the summer of 1956 after his first year at the University of Illinois College of Medicine. He had come to stay with a friend and to find a summer job, and he heard there were jobs available at the Rochester State Hospital. As he walked out to the state hospital, the new Olmsted Community Hospital caught his eye, and he stopped to talk with Mr. Linville. He was offered a job on the spot running the autoclave and cleaning the emergency room. Dr. Peyla met Dr. Verby and learned about the Olmsted Medical Group, and he also met his future wife Betty Anderson, a nurse anesthetist. He returned the next summer to serve as Olmsted Community Hospital's first extern. The externship program gave medical students exposure to real-life practice by having them accompany doctors as they visited patients, and it allowed the medical staff to engage in some teaching.

---

[108] Now behind the main clinic building next to the rear parking area.

Dr. Peyla finished medical school at Illinois, interned in Fresno, California, spent two years in the Air Force, and then returned to Rochester for a pediatrics residency at Mayo Clinic. As Dr. Peyla neared the end of his residency, Dr. Verby approached him about starting a pediatrics department at the Olmsted Medical Group and asked him to bring along another pediatrician. Dr. Peyla recruited Dr. James Hartfield, a native of Houston, Texas, and they were hired to start in 1964.[109] Dr. Peyla became very popular with both patients and their parents, and he was the heart of the pediatrics department for more than 41 years. Dr. Hartfield was called to active duty in the Air Force in August 1966, but returned to the Olmsted Medical Group two years later. He was active in the community, heading the Boy Scout council and serving on the Rochester School Board from 1977 through 1985. He also served as the Olmsted Medical Group's medical director from 1974 through 1985.

The hiring of the pediatricians created a new space problem, so another addition to the Hillcrest office was built. In July 1964, the doctors were divided evenly between the two offices, with Drs. Verby, Brodhun, Bennett, Campbell, Field, Burich, and Peyla at Third Avenue and Drs. Wente, Fluegel, Doyle, Kaese, Pougiales, Sander, and Hartfield at Hillcrest.

As the Olmsted Medical Group grew larger and was divided between its two locations, the doctors and support staff had less interaction at work and socially. To reduce the isolation and to promote camaraderie, the Olmsted Medical Group began organizing social events. For a few winters, it held a family skating party at the Mayo Auditorium, Rochester's only indoor ice rink at the time. After a hiatus of a few decades, these resumed at the Rochester Recreation Center. In the summers, the Olmsted Medical Group hosted family picnics at the Silver Lake pavilion, which became a long-lasting tradition. By the late 1980s, the Olmsted Medical Group outgrew the Silver Lake location, and after trying out several nearby parks, the picnic was moved to the Skyline water park south of town for several years as a daylong event. The picnic was replaced in 2002 with the Olmsted Medical Center's Day at the Movies, which has proved to be very popular with the staff and their families. In the late 1960s, the Olmsted Medical Group's doctors and their spouses started a holiday tradition of progressive dinners with each course hosted at a different home. By 1972, the Olmsted Medical Group was too large for such an intimate event, and the dinners were

---

[109] Peyla, T.L., Interview, Sep. 18, 2008.

moved to Michael's restaurant through the mid-1980s, when the restaurant, too, could no longer accommodate the increasing number of staff. The event then moved to hotel ballrooms for an annual January holiday party that became a tradition and the precursor of today's organization-wide holiday party at the Mayo Civic Center.

Much of 1965 was taken up with issues of growth, with the Olmsted Medical Group planning another addition to the Hillcrest office. Additional land north of the Third Avenue building was now available for $20,000 per acre, and a nursing home company was interested in building on part of it if the Olmsted Medical Group stayed there. Mr. Mills, the management consultant, was again asked to review the Olmsted Medical Group. He reported that the Olmsted Medical Group was financially extended and advised against taking on any new building projects for a few years until the financial position improved. Mr. Mills again noted low productivity and advised tracking each doctor's production and implementing an incentive bonus rather than paying equal salaries. His recommendations were controversial for a few years, but were gradually implemented in various forms. Mr. Mills also advised against adding more medical specialties. A few of the doctors had wanted to do that—and time would support them.

In January 1964, the Olmsted Medical Group made its first profit-sharing contribution of $13,300, which was invested in savings certificates in two different banks since deposit insurance covered only $10,000 at each bank. In September 1965, Dr. Wente and Mr. Wilkus reported to the Olmsted Medical Group board that they had discussed with Mr. Plunkett and their accountant the possibility of having the profit-sharing trust purchase the Olmsted Medical Group buildings, but had been advised not to pursue that at the time.

* * *

Lack of space at the Olmsted Community Hospital continued to be an issue, and in January 1965, Dr. Wente urged the hospital medical staff to present a unified front and push the hospital and county boards on the hospital expansion. The staff passed a resolution to present to the county board on April 5. The following week, the county board resolved to issue up to $450,000 in general revenue bonds to finance an addition, and in August, the bonds were sold to the First National Bank of Rochester. Ellerbe continued to be the architects.

The Olmsted Community Hospital medical service was formed in September 1965. Rather than continue the practice of having all the doctors make rounds at the hospital every morning, one internist and one general practitioner worked at the hospital for one month at a time to care for all the Olmsted Medical Group's medical patients regardless of who was the primary physician. A medical service physician was in the hospital at all times during the day and on call at night. This new system was much more efficient and offered the advantage of having a doctor in the hospital all day. While individual doctors still had the option of caring for their own patients, most quickly adopted the new system. This evolved into the present full-time hospitalist model, which has been widely adopted throughout the country as a means of improving hospital care.

Momentum picked up in 1966 on all fronts. On March 7, representatives of Ellerbe discussed the hospital expansion program with the county board. On March 22, the hospital staff was informed that the plans were awaiting the final approval by the U.S. Public Health Service, which was needed to secure the Hill-Burton funding. In May, the county gave a portion of the hospital property to the city to build a maintenance garage.[110] On November 15, the county board approved the plans and specifications and authorized bids for construction. Bids were opened on December 20, and on January 3, 1967, the contracts were awarded subject to approval by the U.S. Department of Health, Education, and Welfare. The bids were almost $200,000 less than expected—a pleasant surprise.

An interesting issue for the medical staff in 1966 was that of smoking by patients and visitors in the hospital. The staff recommended to the administration that smoking be limited to private rooms and only with the consent of the patient and his or her doctor, but no action was taken. This issue would continue to light up occasionally over the next years.

* * *

At the Olmsted Medical Group, the building partnership sold the Third Avenue buildings to the Profit-Sharing Trust June 1, 1966, for $246,000. The trust assumed the $121,770 mortgage. It also paid the Olmsted Medical Group $124,230 for its interest in the Hillcrest property, which allowed the

---

[110] The Olmsted Medical Center is now buying back the property for $1.2 million.

Olmsted Medical Group to pay off all but $30,000 of its debt. The board instructed Dr. Wente to negotiate the purchase of the land to the north of the main office as soon as possible. The purchase of 3.53 acres from the Graham estate by the trust was completed as of December 31, and a building committee was appointed: Dr. Verby, chair; Dr. Bennett; and Mr. Wilkus.

Since its beginning, the Olmsted Medical Group had encouraged participation in medical organizations and staff education. It paid medical society dues and provided funds for continuing medical education on an ad hoc basis. The board was ahead of its time in 1966 when it established an allowance for each physician to budget his or her own expenses—a practice that is common in medical groups today.

Another event in 1966 was a visit to the Olmsted Medical Group by Drs. Leonard Kurland and Fred Nobrega from the Mayo Clinic department of biostatistics. They were starting a longitudinal epidemiologic study of the residents of Olmsted County to be known as the Rochester Epidemiology Project, which would become the world's largest such repository of medical data and the source of thousands of important studies. Since the Mayo Clinic and the Olmsted Medical Group provided practically all the healthcare for Olmsted County residents, the researchers wanted to include the Olmsted Medical Group's patient records in their database. After meeting with the Olmsted Medical Group's board, they met with the Olmsted Community Hospital staff on several occasions to discuss modifications in the records that would help with data retrieval and to encourage a higher autopsy rate. Dr. Kurland's staff abstracted the Olmsted Medical Group's patient records back to the first day of Dr. Wente's practice in 1949.

The first research project to involve Olmsted Medical Group patients was proposed in September 1966, when Dr. Norman Keith of the Mayo Clinic presented a study of congestive heart failure and enlisted the hospital medical staff's participation. This started a long era of cooperation in medical research that continues to this day through the Olmsted Medical Center research department. In addition, Dr. Jack Whisnant, chair of the Mayo Regional Medical Outreach Committee, approached the Olmsted Medical Group about cooperating with a regional medical center study, and Drs. Verby and Campbell were assigned to act as liaisons.

The Olmsted Medical Group was not satisfied with the accuracy of tests sent to a large outside laboratory and discussed the problem with Dr. Whisnant. He informed the Olmsted Medical Group that Mayo Clinic would be willing to do some laboratory and other procedures for them and that he would do in-hospital neurologic consultations. This was the first formal arrangement between the Olmsted Medical Group and Mayo Clinic, and a good example of the cooperative and collaborative relationship that the two organizations still enjoy.

* * *

Construction of the hospital addition started on March 3, 1967. It would add 30 beds, bringing the total 80. The major part was the construction of a large wing on the west side of the building to house obstetrical services. This wing had a basement, which the original building did not. A second elevator was installed next to the first, and the renovation expanded the cafeteria and provided administrative offices. A small addition on the east side enlarged the laboratory and sterile supply area, provided locker rooms for surgical staff, and created a postoperative recovery room. The new elevator did not solve the problem of patients having to go through the front lobby to X-ray or surgery, though. An open house was held on Sunday, May 5, 1968, to celebrate the renovation. The new facility made it possible for the hospital's obstetrics department to deliver 100 more babies during the next year.

When the Olmsted Community Hospital opened in 1955, there had been talk of establishing a program to train practical nurses, but it was thought to be too complicated in the midst of opening a new hospital. By 1967, conditions permitted such a program, and a training program was established in 1967 by the Rochester School District, which ran the vocational-technical program until 1969. The hospital became the primary training site for the new licensed practical nurse program, which continues today. This began a hospital tradition of providing education for a variety of health professionals including pharmacists, social workers, and nurses, who to this day continue to receive part of their training at the Olmsted Medical Center.

* * *

The Olmsted Medical Group had more expansion plans of its own, and invited Harold Westin to visit. Mr. Westin, an architect and engineer who had been a professor at the University of Minnesota, was known for pursuing the case that made it legal to have design-build contracts in the state. Previously, architects and builders had to be separate entities as the architect supervised the builder. Mr. Westin had done a lot of work using this method in the Twin Cities, including the Nicollet and Earl clinics in St. Paul. He visited Rochester in April 1967 to look at the Olmsted Medical Group and advise whether a major addition or an entirely new building was the better solution to the ongoing space crunch. He recommended building a new structure, and by November produced a design, but the building committee turned down the proposal and looked elsewhere.

Dr. Verby had taken a three-month sabbatical to study the practice of family medicine in Europe in the summer of 1967, and Dr. Burich replaced him as chair of the building committee. After turning down Mr. Westin's proposal, the committee worked for a time with three firms in Madison, Wisconsin, one of which flew them around the country in a private jet to look at other medical buildings. But the committee didn't care for these companies, either, and went back to Mr. Westin the following summer with some of Dr. Burich's design ideas. They looked at more of Mr. Westin's work, and he developed an acceptable plan, even though it was $50,000 more than their budget. Financing was complicated by Minnesota's 8% interest limit at a time of rising inflation and increasing interest rates. The Olmsted Medical Group worked out a deal with Lutheran Brotherhood for a $725,000 loan for the building at 8% interest. Lutheran Brotherhood bought the land for $100,000 and leased it back for $12,000 a year, making an effective rate of 8.5%.

Ground was broken for the new home of the Olmsted Medical Group on Wednesday, August 20, 1969, just a little more than 20 years after Dr. Wente had opened his tiny office over Lawler's Dry Cleaners. In the interim, the Hillcrest office was remodeled to provide four more exam rooms and more waiting space.

Meanwhile, in July 1967, Dr. James Garber had joined the Olmsted Medical Group's internal medicine department. He was from Albert Lea, received his medical degree from the University of Minnesota, and completed his residency at the Mayo Clinic, where he was regarded as one of the stars of its program. He remained with the Olmsted Medical Group for his entire career and filled several key roles including that of medical director. In addition to continuing to expand its medical staff, the Olmsted Medical

Group also invested in innovative technology by acquiring a 90-second automatic X-ray processor and renting its first pagers, rather clunky gadgets, from the telephone company.

Dr. Neal Olson, a graduate of the Mayo Clinic pediatrics program, joined Dr. Peyla and Dr. Hartfield several days after Dr. Hartfield returned from the Air Force. Dr. Olson was a native of Rochester, whose father was the O in O&B Shoes, and he was a patient of Dr. Wente as a child, which made Dr. Wente feel old. Dr. Olson had planned to take an allergy fellowship, and Dr. Peyla had tried to convince him to join the Olmsted Medical Group immediately when he finished his pediatric training in 1967 and do the fellowship after Dr. Hartfield's return. But Dr. Olson did the allergy fellowship and then joined the Olmsted Medical Group afterwards in October 1968. The three pediatricians developed a bustling practice that included many children of Mayo Clinic physicians.

Dr. Robert Konicek also joined the Olmsted Medical Group in 1968. A native of Prairie du Chien, he had graduated from Marquette University and its medical school, and was practicing alone in Tomah, Wisconsin. He had let it be known that he was interested in joining a group, so the Wentes visited him and his wife, Trudy. The two couples hit it off immediately. Dr. Konicek was a great addition—experienced and used to working hard, he could handle anything and was always the first to volunteer. He was also a man of many hobbies—woodworking, welding, bee keeping, gardening, square dancing, and more—and had a great sense of humor.

By now, Dr. Wente had been the leader of the Olmsted Medical Group for nearly 20 years and was generally respected by the members for his business acumen. His practice had gravitated toward acute illness, and he was leaving the serious cases to the recently educated and more specialized doctors. He thought that perhaps the Olmsted Medical Group should have a medical director or chief of professional services to deal with medical practice issues. The board discussed the idea in May 1968, and, after further consideration, decided to offer the position to Dr. Garber, who agreed to start in January 1969. He was in charge of physician recruiting and dealing with any physician or medical issues that might arise.

In addition to his European sabbatical, Dr. Verby was becoming more interested in academic matters and was working part-time with the Rochester

Epidemiology Project on a study of thyroiditis. At the July 1968 Olmsted Medical Group board meeting, Dr. Verby announced that Dr. Ben Fuller, who was developing the new family practice department at the University of Minnesota, wanted to meet to discuss a program of medical student externships throughout the state and to obtain the Olmsted Medical Group's participation. Then in November, Dr. Verby[111] announced his resignation from the Olmsted Medical Group to take a position at the university heading the Rural Physician Associate Program, in which medical students spend nine months to a year working with physicians in rural or small-town practices.

In February 1969, the Olmsted Medical Group joined the American Association of Medical Clinics, now the American Medical Group Association. The association provided some group insurance benefits, but it was much more valuable as an educational tool for the Olmsted Medical Group's leadership. Both the formal conference presentations and the networking opportunities would have major impacts. The Olmsted Medical Group's large number of general practitioners, which was very unusual for multispecialty groups at the time, and its proximity to the Mayo Clinic made it an instant curiosity and Dr. Wente a star attraction at the association meetings.[112]

By this time, the Olmsted Medical Group had outgrown its Subchapter S organizational structure. If all physicians were to become shareholders, they would need to create a regular professional corporation to be taxed as a unit rather than as individuals. This was discussed throughout the year, and incorporation under the new structure was completed as of January 1, 1970. The clinical organization had also been an issue throughout 1969. The Olmsted Medical Group wanted to maintain unity by avoiding separation into individually managed departments, yet the growth of each specialty raised divisive and competing interests. A committee of section representatives who were not board members was formed in January to deal with such issues, and Dr. Garber met with the sections as well. The sections led an ambiguous existence for several years until the Olmsted Medical Group acknowledged the reality of its increasing size by recognizing departments and appointing chairs for them.

---

[111] Dr. Verby died on October 23, 2007.
[112] He chaired the AAMC Committee on Health Care planning in the mid-1970s and spoke at the 1976 meeting on "Family Practice—Integration into Multispecialty Settings."

At the end of 1969, Dr. Field left to join the faculty of the University of Nebraska. By the 1960s, fewer physicians were entering general practice, and to help meet modern needs, the specialty of family practice was established, with three-year residencies and certification by the American Board of Family Practice, which was created in 1969. Experienced general practitioners could be certified by taking an examination. The University of Minnesota's family practice residency was one of the original 15 nationwide that were accredited in December 1969. Dr. Wente was in the first group to pass the two-day certification exam in early 1970.[113]

Continuing a Olmsted Medical Group method of recruiting, the random drop-in visit, Dr. Nancy Grubbs stopped by the Olmsted Medical Group one day in 1969. A graduate of the University of Missouri College of Medicine, she had completed her internship and was in Rochester while her husband, Larry, completed an internship at the Mayo Clinic. He had been a veterinarian, but developed allergies to animal dander and switched to human medicine, completing his medical degree at Missouri where the couple had met. Dr. Grubbs started work at the Olmsted Medical Group "temporarily" in 1970, but, rather than leaving when her husband finished his training program at Mayo Clinic, as had so many other residents' wives, Larry joined the Olmsted Medical Group the next October and stayed for 35 years. The Grubbses were the first of several physician couples in the Olmsted Medical Group.

In January 1970, Dr. Wente had reached the end of his tolerance with the smoking problems at the Hillcrest office, especially in the obstetrics waiting area, and he made it the state's first smoke-free medical facility. The Guest House, a treatment facility for chemically dependent Catholic priests, had recently opened just northeast of town and Dr. Garber became its medical director, beginning a long career in the field of addiction medicine.

Dr. Richard Christiana, another mainstay of the Olmsted Medical Group, was born in New York and raised in San Jose, California. He graduated from San Jose State University and the University of Utah School of Medicine. After his internship, he served two years in the Navy, mostly in Guam. He came to Rochester in the summer of 1968 for an orthopedics residency at

[113] Angela Curran, Center for the History of Family Medicine; Wente memoirs; Wente papers, Olmsted Medical Center Archive.

the Mayo Clinic. Having a couple of months before his program started, he worked with Dr. Dale Hawk in St. Charles. After a year and a half of orthopedics, Dr. Christiana switched to radiology and then dropped out of that in July 1970. He worked with Dr. Hawk again for about three months, and then joined the Olmsted Medical Group on October 12, 1970, just in time to work for two or three weeks in the Third Avenue building before moving to the new building. Dr. Christiana quickly developed a devoted following, heavy in IBMers and their families. He always described his patients to other doctors as "very nice." Seven years later, Dr. Christiana decided to go back into radiology, but he soon realized it was too separated from the ongoing patient care that he loved, and he returned to the Olmsted Medical Group within a few days.

* * *

While the Olmsted Medical Group continued to grow, the Olmsted Community Hospital lost most of its other physicians to retirement or to other hospitals closer to their offices. By the end of 1968, there were only three active staff physicians who were not members of the Olmsted Medical Group—Dr. Risser, Dr. Wellner, and Dr. C.W. Baars, a psychiatrist in private practice. By 1974, Dr. Risser was the only physician at the hospital who was not a member of the Olmsted Medical Group.

In March 1970, the hospital medical staff passed a resolution declaring that cigarette machines in the hospital lobby should be removed, that the auxiliary should stop selling cigarettes from their cart, and that there should be no smoking in patient rooms—only in the lobbies. The resolution was sent to both the administration and the auxiliary, but was not implemented.

The main deficiency after the hospital addition opened was equipment for the radiology department. Dr. Corrigan had been complaining for some time that the equipment was obsolete and frequently inoperative. The medical staff passed a resolution in June 1969 supporting the need for a new X-ray machine. In May 1970, Dr. Corrigan reported that a lease-purchase agreement had been arranged for a new General Electric machine. The hospital was short of cash and went to the county board for a loan. On November 17, 1970, the county board passed a resolution that began, "WHEREAS Olmsted County in the creation of the Olmsted Community Hospital board invested it with broad powers and diversified duties and responsibilities in the high hope of the Olmsted Community Hospital being self-sufficient without need for a partially sustaining County levy to augment its receipts," and so on for four more "whereases" about how the hospital was, is, and evermore shall not cost the county any more money. The result was that the county loaned the hospital $48,610 at 0.5% monthly interest to be repaid within five years. A new X-ray machine was installed the following April, although it did not have the capabilities that Dr. Corrigan originally requested.

* * *

As the Olmsted Medical Group's new building was being planned, there was talk of building a Kmart store to its north if the city would agree to extend Ninth Street eastward from Third Avenue to Broadway. The Olmsted Medical Group opposed this because it felt that Kmart did not fit the residential neighborhood, and it was concerned about the increased traffic and the cost of the street expansion. The Kmart was eventually built as planned at this location and has proved to be an additional attraction to Olmsted Medical Group patients for shopping and pharmacy needs before or after their appointments.

The new building provided for space for a pharmacy to be leased by Carl Ruffalo, and an optical shop to be operated by Stan Gibbons. There were two particularly innovative features in the new building. The first was that the building was to be only the second in the country after the St. Louis Park Clinic to have a German-designed "Tele-Lift" system, small cars that run on tracks between the departments, up walls and between floors to carry patient records and other material. The cars had more capacity than a tube system, and records could be kept flat rather than rolled up. This system is still in use at the Rochester Southeast Clinic building. The second innovation was that the floors—other than those of the lowest levels—were constructed of gypsum panels in a steel framework coated with mastic to make a smooth, firm surface. The mastic did not adhere properly, though, and these floors continued to be a problem for 15 years until they were covered with concrete when the third floor was added. One-third of the lower level was left unfinished, with a sand floor for future installation of utilities. Moving day was October 30, and the new building opened for business on Monday, November 2, 1970. An open house on December 6 attracted 2,000 visitors to tour the new facility.

The 15 years between 1955 and 1970 were filled with intense activities at the hospital and Olmsted Medical Group that had lasting consequences. The hospital proved to be very popular and successful, necessitating an expansion. The county board repeatedly refused to appoint a medical staff physician to the hospital board. The Olmsted Medical Group hired a professional administrator, changed its corporate structure to accommodate more growth and equity, employed a medical director, and settled into a permanent location. A profit-sharing trust was developed and funded, and Dr. Wente declared an end to smoking at the Hillcrest office.

As 1970 drew to a close, IBM had grown to 4,200 employees; Rochester's population had grown to more than 52,000; the Olmsted Community Hospital had 80 beds and bassinets; and the Olmsted Medical Group had 19 doctors and counting. That growth would continue—bringing more growing pains. There would be more innovation and some missed opportunities—and certainly plenty of interesting times.

Chapter 5
Change and Opportunities

On the ground, the Olmsted Medical Group continued its success along the same trajectory. In the air, changes were swirling, a mixture of good and bad ideas. Some came to fruition, and others did not. It wasn't always the good that did or the bad that did not.

One of the better ideas discussed was accreditation by the Accreditation Association for Ambulatory Health Care (AAAHC). The Olmsted Medical Group applied for accreditation and in November 1971 a survey team spent two days examining the organization, facilities, and practices, and it became one of the early groups to be accredited.

Another move that proved to be valuable to the Olmsted Medical Group was hiring retired Mayo Clinic physicians. Among the physicians who joined the Olmsted Medical Group in 1972 was Dr. Thomas T. Myers, who had developed the specialty of vein surgery at the Mayo Clinic. When he reached 65, he was required to retire from Mayo Clinic, but he did not want to retire from surgery or to move away from Rochester. He began working part-time at the Olmsted Medical Group, operating one day a week and spending a half-day or two in the office. Dr. Harry Swedlund, an allergist, and Dr. Charles Dicken, a dermatologist, were other Mayo Clinic retirees who made major contributions to the Olmsted Medical Group through several years of service.

The Olmsted Medical Group felt that it needed its own radiologist rather than continue to contract with Dr. Corrigan, who was still working at the Olmsted Community Hospital. Dr. Wente informed Dr. Corrigan that the Olmsted Medical Group was going to employ its own radiologist and offered him the first opportunity. While he would have preferred the status quo, Dr. Corrigan realized that he could not successfully compete with the Olmsted Medical Group and accepted the offer.

Another good idea and an opportunity to collaborate with Mayo Clinic occurred when Dr. Robert Schrantz, the Olmsted Community Hospital's pathologist, decided to leave. The Olmsted Medical Group first worked with Mr. Linville to find a replacement who could meet the needs of both organizations, but it was unsuccessful. After talks with the Mayo Clinic pathology department, Mayo Clinic assumed supervision, on July 1, 1972, of both the Olmsted Medical Group and Olmsted Community Hospital laboratories with Dr. Michael O'Sullivan in charge, assuring that the labs met the same standards as Mayo Clinic's own. Mayo Clinic performed the surgical pathology with frozen sections performed at Rochester Methodist Hospital.

One idea that did not come to fruition was the suggestion that Rochester's obstetrical services be combined into one unit. Mayo Clinic was planning to move its obstetrical unit out of St. Marys Hospital because of conflicts over performing post-partum tubal ligations in the Catholic hospital. Because the number of deliveries at St. Marys was insufficient for their obstetrics training program requirements, Mayo Clinic residents were required to obtain part of their training at Cook County Hospital in Chicago in order to gain enough experience. Two proposals were considered for combining obstetrics—a freestanding unit adjacent to the Olmsted Community Hospital or rotating Mayo Clinic residents through the hospital. Other possible collaborations discussed with Mayo Clinic included coordination of the care of nursing home patients and a suggestion by Dr. Wente that the county's public health director work part-time for the county and be a professor at the new Mayo Medical School. This idea was not implemented either.

By 1972, Dr. Wente was envisioning a system of family practice clinics in area towns within 30 miles or so linked to the Olmsted Medical Group, which would then be linked to Mayo Clinic, providing a rational continuous process of care. This idea anticipated the Mayo Health System by two decades. He applied for a grant from the Northlands Regional Medical Program[114] for "A Pilot Demonstration Project to Develop a System for Bringing to Rural Communities a Complete Range of Quality Primary and Secondary Health Services that are Group Practice Oriented."

Dr. Wente did not get the grant, but he proceeded anyway. He first approached Dr. Risser in Stewartville, who had no interest in changing his practice or associating with the Olmsted Medical Group. Dr. Wente then considered opening a family practice clinic in St. Charles, where Dr. Dale Hawk was practicing. From a small town in Ohio, Dr. Hawk graduated from Kent State and Hahneman Medical College. After practicing near Cleveland for about five years, he moved to St. Charles in 1957 to join another new

---

[114] Olmsted Medical Group Board Minutes, July 11, 1972; Wente papers

physician, Dr. Sam McHutchison, in a new clinic the town was building. They bought the building, but after Dr. McHutchison moved to St. Paul in 1963, Dr. Hawk was unable to find a long-term partner. He was known to be very personable and a friend of the Olmsted Medical Group's doctors.

At that time, the residents of St. Charles, which is just over the county line in Winona County, did most of their business in Winona, the county seat. It was hard to convince them to use the Olmsted Community Hospital, even though it was a bit closer than Winona was. At some point, telephone calls from St. Charles to Rochester became free instead of long distance, and almost overnight St. Charles turned 180 degrees to face Rochester rather than Winona—an interesting lesson in economics. Dr. Wente and Mr. Wilkus approached Dr. Hawk in June 1972, and he agreed to join the Olmsted Medical Group in 1973. The Olmsted Medical Group agreed to lease Dr. Hawk's building and to make some improvements. Dr. Hawk had an option to leave the Olmsted Medical Group within two years if he was not happy with the arrangement.[115]

Other ideas and issues were being discussed at the Olmsted Community Hospital. In a hospital staff educational session in 1971, Dr. Kaese talked about the changing and increasing indications for cesarean section and the increasing demand for surgical sterilization, especially tubal ligation. The next year, the state medical association reported that there was no law requiring consultation with a second physician before sterilization,[116] then a standard practice which made it more difficult for women to obtain the procedure. On January 22, 1973, the U.S. Supreme Court ruled on Roe versus Wade. If tubal ligation was controversial, abortion was even more so. The Olmsted Medical Group quickly stated that it felt no obligation to perform abortions on request, but would continue its policy of performing an abortion only if the mother's life were in danger. St. Marys Hospital banned abortions entirely, while the Mayo Clinic said only that "each case would be evaluated with … sound medical judgment."[117]

With the St. Charles clinic off to a good start, Dr. Wente suggested looking for another opportunity, perhaps in Kasson. However, Mr. Wilkus received

---

[115] Wente memoirs; Hawk, D.J., Interview, Oct. 22, 2007.
[116] This had been a common practice as sterilization is usually permanent and some people had moral issues concerning it.
[117] *Rochester Post-Bulletin*, Feb. 2, 1973, p. 19.

a call for help from Hayfield, where the town's only doctor had left. The Austin Clinic had filled in, but now it was losing its doctor who had been working in Hayfield and did not plan to replace him. An agreement was reached for the Olmsted Medical Group to lease the town's clinic building, and the its second branch clinic was opened on September 1, 1973.

In December 1973, the Olmsted Medical Group's board of directors decided to expand the medical director's duties to strengthen physician leadership. The medical director would be in charge of the clinical aspects of the practice, just as Mr. Wilkus was in charge of the business side. At the same time, Dr. Garber's work as medical director had become an increasing burden. He had no time set aside for this work and had a very busy practice, especially when he was on hospital service. Dr. Hartfield, on the other hand, had a less busy practice and an interest in management. Dr. Wente asked him to take the job, with neither of them knowing exactly what the job would shape up to be. Fortuitously, the 25th anniversary meeting of the American Association of Medical Clinics was just a couple of months later. The organization changed its name to the American Group Practice Association and hosted a meeting of medical directors. That led to the formation of the American Academy of Medical Directors, which is now the American College of Physician Executives (ACPE) and active in developing management courses for physician leaders. The ACPE became a valuable asset for Olmsted Medical Group leaders, many of whom received management training through its courses. It would provide a life-altering experience for Dr. Hartfield, who became a charter member.

To enhance physician leadership, the Olmsted Medical Group board decided to formalize the clinical departments. Dr. Hartfield took on this task, along with developing a systems and procedures manual and organizing a professional services committee. At the same time, the board's agendas had become overcrowded and the meetings often lasted until midnight. Dr. Wente thought that an executive committee composed of the president, medical director, and administrator could handle much of the board business. The board somewhat reluctantly agreed; they liked the alternative of interminable board meetings less. The occasional name changes between executive committee, management group, and administrative team reflected varying attitudes about the role and scope of this committee over the years, and it is now known as the board executive committee.

* * *

Such was the state of the Olmsted Medical Group in 1974 when I joined it. Like Dr. Wente when he opened his practice on 1949, I had no idea what I would be getting into and how the future would unfold. My wife, Karen, and I arrived at the Holiday Inn South in Rochester on Sunday evening, January 6, 1974. When the sun rose, the temperature was 30 degrees below zero, and I wondered what I was doing here. The oldest of six children, I was born in Evansville, Indiana on July 1, 1940, and was mostly raised in the country a few miles out of town. My father was a commercial artist who became the design director of a major printing company, and my mother was a special education teacher. They were active in the civil rights movement, especially concerning open housing. They would be honored by the local Ku Klux Klan with a cross burning on their front yard on Martin Luther King Day in 1979.

I was a debater throughout high school and college and graduated from DePauw University. Early in my second year at Northwestern University Medical School, I was eating supper in the Passavant Hospital cafeteria when I met the most perfect creature I had ever seen. Karen Sandberg was a second-year nursing student, very blonde and 100% Swedish, I learned. We were married in her home church in Rockford, Illinois, a little less than two years later. After medical school, I stayed at Northwestern for six years of surgical training and then spent two years in the Army Medical Corps at Fort Campbell.

Early in the autumn of my second year in the Army, Karen and I began to look for a place to spend the rest of our lives. We visited medical groups from Fredericksburg, Virginia, in an arc through Tennessee, Kentucky, Indiana, and Illinois to Green Bay, Wisconsin, without finding what we wanted. At a surgical meeting, I met a prominent surgeon from Fond du Lac, Wisconsin, who invited me to visit after Christmas. I learned that Dr. Strobel, a surgeon at the Mankato Clinic, was planning to retire, so I decided to visit there as well. I would never have considered Siberia, Antarctica, or Minnesota, but one of my sisters married a man from St. Paul and lived there for more than eight years without freezing to death, so I knew Minnesota was habitable at least that far north. I had received information from the Olmsted Medical Group, but thought Rochester had more than enough surgeons already. Dr. John Tinker,[118] an anesthesiologist at Fort Campbell, was getting out of the

---

[118] Later head of the Anesthesia Department at the University of Iowa and now chairman at the University of Nebraska.

Army a few months ahead of me and was going on staff at the Mayo Clinic. He said that he had heard good things about the Olmsted Medical Group and said that, as long as Karen and I were going right by it on the way to Mankato, I should stop and have a look. So on our way to Mankato and Fond du Lac, we dropped off the kids (our first two) in Rockford with their grandparents and kept going north. Driving across Interstate 90 in January was not especially inspiring.

On Monday morning, although it was 30 degrees below zero, there was no wind, and there had been a heavy frost. The sun came out, and the trees and wires sparkled like fairyland. It was beautiful, and I thought, "This is as cold is it ever gets. I can handle this." They didn't tell me about minus 75 degree wind chills. I called Frank Wilkus for directions to the Olmsted Medical Group clinic. He said to turn right at the first "semaphore" after Highway 14. I had never heard a traffic light called a "semaphore," but we somehow arrived. Sally Hartfield took Karen on a tour of the town and schools while Dr. Hartfield, Dr. Wente, and Mr. Wilkus gave me a tour of the main clinic and the Olmsted Community Hospital. I was impressed with the Olmsted Medical Group's organization—it was many times better than any other I had seen. The building was first rate, spacious, well lighted, and well designed. I also liked the people I met.

The hospital was less impressive but seemed adequate, and it was as good as or better than others that I had visited and a step up from the termite-infested hospital at Fort Campbell. I talked with Mr. Linville and explained my interest in vascular surgery, but he didn't understand why I should do vascular surgery and wasn't interested in buying the necessary $2,000 worth of instruments, even though one operation would have returned the investment. I met Karen late in the afternoon to travel to Mankato. She informed me that she was moving to Rochester and that, if I wished, I could come too. We learned that Dr. Strobel in Mankato wasn't retiring that week after all—he vacillated for a few years before taking up pig farming full-time. After a brief return to Rockford, Karen and I visited Fond du Lac and easily decided that it was not the right practice for me.

We came back to Rochester three days after the first visit, and I signed on the dotted line. My salary was $2,000 less than the going rate—the Olmsted Medical Group bought the vascular surgery instruments and donated them to the hospital. Ironically, when we moved into our new home in Rochester on July 12, the temperature set a record high of 103 degrees. We also had a record early frost that year—in August! Our first winter in Rochester brought the "blizzard of the century," with about one inch of snow and another of South Dakota topsoil, along with a record low barometric pressure. And that spring, the first three times the temperature reached 70 degrees, it snowed the next day. Minnesota weather proved to be very interesting.

The surgical practice was interesting too. During my first month, everyone sent me a "welcome case," and I was busy right away. Dr. Sander and especially Dr. Burich taught me how to do orthopedic procedures I hadn't done in residency and gave me a refresher on tonsillectomies, which I hadn't done for several years. I liked the fact that seven members of the Olmsted Medical Group, including me, drove Volkswagen Beetles to work. At a surgical group I had considered joining, the doctors had matching maroon Lincoln Continentals. They also had pretentious houses, and their wives were grande dames of local society, always in the spotlight. Karen and I preferred the atmosphere of Rochester and the Olmsted Medical Group, which was much more informal and collegial. I was shocked, however, to find that in this medical Mecca of the world that newspaper stories promoted the quack cancer drug Laetrile.

* * *

The Olmsted Medical Group continued its course on the leading edge of medical practice by establishing the second patient education department in the state. This department was staffed by Connie DeLorme, PhD, a nutritionist who had taught and done research at the University of Minnesota. Colleen Gau, RN, whose husband was a Mayo Clinic cardiologist, also worked in patient education, especially with heart patients, and she performed a very important service for the hospital in discharge planning, which the hospital itself didn't provide.

Dr. Wente's effort to establish a system of branch clinics in the region stumbled in October when Dr. Hawk decided to disaffiliate his St. Charles practice from the Olmsted Medical Group. Dr. Hawk was used to being his own boss and that of his employees. Mr. Wilkus seemed insensitive to the cultural differences in the small-town clinic, and he and Dr. Hawk had butted heads over a number of issues. Dr. Hawk remained a friend of the Olmsted Medical Group, though, and it provided care for his patients when he was on vacation.

* * *

The Olmsted Community Hospital medical staff again pursued the issue of banning tobacco sales in the hospital after both the Minnesota State Medical Association and the Minnesota Hospital Association passed resolutions against tobacco sales in hospitals in 1974. Once again, the medical staff sent letters to both the administration and auxiliary. The administrator left it up to the auxiliary, which finally decided to discontinue tobacco sales.

Another issue for the hospital staff involved the anesthesia department. The Joint Commission on Accreditation of Hospitals now required that physician directors be appointed to oversee hospital anesthesia departments. At that time, the Olmsted Community Hospital anesthesia department was staffed by nurse anesthetists. They were supervised by the operating surgeon in each case, but there was no overall physician direction for the department. It was thought that Mayo Clinic would be willing to provide a physician director, just as it was providing a physician laboratory director. In the interim, I was appointed to the position. I had had a month of anesthesia training as an intern, but mainly no one else wanted the job and I was the junior surgeon. The Mayo Clinic anesthesiology department did not have enough staff to assist us, so I remained chief of anesthesia until the Olmsted Medical Group hired its first anesthesiologist more than 10 years later. The next year, the Joint Commission added similar requirements for chiefs of medicine and surgery. Dr. Neal Olson was appointed to the first position, and I was appointed chief of surgery.

Mr. Linville retired as administrator of the Olmsted Community Hospital in 1974 at the age of 72 after twenty years in the position. He was widely praised for his stewardship in keeping the hospital profitable.[119] The Olmsted Medical Group doctors, while appreciating the financial performance of the hospital, had had a number of disagreements with him and looked forward to working with his successor.

* * *

It was not only internal issues that led to changes and challenges in the Olmsted Medical Group and the Olmsted Community Hospital. In the

---

[119] *Rochester Post-Bulletin*, Dec. 30, 1974.

early 1970s, medicine was assaulted from all sides. There was serious inflation in the general economy, which had resulted in price controls for a few years. Price controls continued in force for medical services after they were lifted for other businesses, and the costs of providing care continued to escalate. When the controls were eventually lifted, there followed several years of sharp increases in costs, with employees' salaries and fees being adjusted by several percent twice yearly. Olmsted Medical Group doctors were uncomfortable with the higher fees and often undercharged or didn't charge at all for patient visits, which impaired financial performance. A national malpractice crisis struck at about that time, with a sudden upsurge in lawsuits and high-dollar verdicts. The Olmsted Medical Group's insurance premiums jumped more than 60% in 1974 and 50% more in 1975. The Olmsted Medical Group changed insurers twice to find affordable rates. The Olmsted Medical Group received another surprise when Congress passed the Employee Retirement Income and Security Act of 1974 (ERISA). One provision made it illegal for profit-sharing trusts to own the employer's buildings, which struck at the heart of the financing for the Olmsted Medical Group's new building. The Olmsted Medical Group had 10 years in which to comply with the new law, and its attorneys thought that it was possible it could receive an exemption from the U.S. Department of Labor. At any rate, the Olmsted Medical Group was advised to postpone action on this issue.

The cost of the Medicare program had been grossly underestimated when legislation was passed in 1965. When the true cost became evident, the government began a campaign to reduce Medicare spending with a variety of programs that reduced payments to the providers of medical care. Three early programs were health maintenance organizations (HMOs), professional services review organizations (PSROs), and health systems agencies (HSAs). HMOs paid physicians a flat rate for caring for all of a patient's healthcare needs, and the physicians were often responsible for the costs of the care they did not provide themselves but referred to other physicians. This responsibility of physicians for costs that they could not control was the fatal flaw.[120] PSROs were organizations of physicians who contracted with the government to review the necessity and quality of care for Medicare patients. HSAs planned for the healthcare needs of areas within a state to reduce duplication of services. Major projects required a certificate of need (CON), which ultimately was seen as ineffective because almost every proposal was approved.

---

[120] Today HMOs rarely use this system of payment.

The first of the cost-control issues to affect the Olmsted Medical Group was HMOs. In mid-1973, Dr. Brodun and Mr. Wilkus attended a symposium on HMO development in Minneapolis, which was becoming a hotbed of HMO activity. In January 1974, there were talks between the Olmsted Medical Group and Mayo Clinic about their relationships, the Olmsted Medical Group's regional expansion plan, HMOs, and PSROs. In June, Mr. Wilkus met with Mr. Robert Fleming, the Mayo Clinic administrator. Mayo Clinic had received a grant to start a PSRO, but did not see the need for an HMO. It felt that group practices could be just as efficient at providing care as HMOs and published a study supporting that opinion.[121] Group Health, a pioneer HMO in St. Paul that employed its own salaried physicians, met with the Olmsted Medical Group's executive committee in August 1974 to discuss cooperation in the Rochester area. While not agreeing to work with them, Dr. Wente thought, "There might be something to be said in the prepayment area." The HMO issue would lie dormant for four or five years, but would return.

About the same time, the Mayo Clinic announced a plan to open a medical school. One of the conditions imposed by the state was that Mayo Clinic also would have to start a family practice residency program. These programs were major changes for Mayo Clinic and would eventually lead to problems for the Olmsted Medical Group.

Dr. Wente was serving as chairman of the American Group Practice Association's North Central Region and was asked to chair a committee on primary care, which was still not a major activity for very many large medical groups. As far back as March 1972, he had been having conversations with Dr. John R. Hodgson, chairman of the Mayo Clinic medical services committee, about creating a better organized system of care in the area, and having the Olmsted Medical Group involved with the new Mayo Medical School and family practice residency.

Dr. Wente proposed that the Olmsted Medical Group be replaced by a non-profit entity that would be separate from the Mayo Clinic but that would work closely with it in providing family practice training for medical students and residents.[122] He spoke to the Olmsted Medical Group board of directors

---

[121] JAMA 247: pp. 806-810 (Feb) 1982.
[122] Wente papers, Olmsted Medical Center Archive.

on November 12, 1974, as it appeared that Mayo Clinic was losing interest in the idea. He talked about the coming changes in American medicine and the need to be concerned "if we are interested in perpetuating what we have tried to build here in Rochester." This was the first explicit reference to the idea of the Olmsted Medical Group's becoming a permanent institution, although its incorporation was a major step in that direction. Dr. Wente also discussed the benefit to the community of working with Mayo Clinic, rather than competing and duplicating efforts. Prophetically, he then stated: "I think that we can compete with the Mayo Clinic no matter what they do, no matter what directions they take. I think we grow stronger when we compete. I think we will grow larger, we will have more problems. I think we will perhaps enjoy a greater independence if we go our own way and compete more directly with them. If that is the decision of the Mayo Clinic eventually, why we will live with that and we will probably end up being a larger and stronger organization."[123]

A liaison committee was established to discuss the Olmsted Medical Group's role in the Mayo Clinic family practice residency program. Dr. Guy Dougherty, who was in charge of developing the program, was enthusiastic about the Olmsted Medical Group's involvement. The committee continued to meet through the next spring. On July 8, 1975, Dr. Dougherty and Dr. Ray Pruitt, the dean of the Mayo Medical School, met with Dr. Wente. They agreed that the residents would split their time equally between Mayo Clinic and the Olmsted Medical Group, and that the Olmsted Medical Group physicians would have faculty appointments.[124] Dr. James Aquilino, a residency-trained family physician who had practiced two years in Elmira, New York, joined the Olmsted Medical Group to lead its portion of the residency program.[125]

Meanwhile, in October 1974, Dr. Wente was contacted by a Kasson organization about starting a Olmsted Medical Group branch clinic there. Dr. Wente thought that it would be a good idea to establish a clinic there jointly with Mayo Clinic and that it would be a good training site for medical students. In June 1974, Dodge County had been declared a federal physician

[123] Olmsted Medical Group Board Minutes, Dec. 17, 1974. Transcript in Wente papers, Olmsted Medical Center Archive.
[124] Olmsted Medical Group Board Minutes, July 8, 1975.
[125] Confirmed by Dr. Aquilino.

shortage area and the Area Health Systems Agency recommended that all the communities in the county work together to develop a single medical center. A group of citizens from the county formed a corporation to build a clinic and nursing home in Dodge Center and an ambulance service to serve the whole county. They applied for a grant and asked the Olmsted Medical Group to operate the clinic. It would be staffed initially by Dr. Mary Ann Kimmel, whose husband was from Dodge Center. The Olmsted Medical Group also applied for a physician from the Health Service Corps to serve in the designated shortage area.

But in August, while the Dodge Center group awaited its grant, the Mayo Clinic announced that it was building a large clinic in Kasson, which would be the base for its new family practice residency. The construction of this clinic also meant that Dodge County would no longer be underserved and that Dodge Center would no longer qualify for a physician through the Health Service Corps. Dr. James Hunt, chairman of Mayo Clinic's internal medicine department, asked Drs. Wente and Garber and Mr. Wilkus to meet with him, Dr. Dougherty, Dr. Hodgson, and Mr. Robert Fleming on September 22. At the beginning of the meeting, Dr. Hunt announced that his department would supervise the family practice residency, that the medical school had nothing to do with it, and that the Olmsted Medical Group would have no role in it. The Olmsted Medical Group, understandably, felt betrayed. This marked a low point in the generally good relations between Mayo Clinic and the Olmsted Medical Group.

The Olmsted-Medical-Group-affiliated Dodge Center Clinic opened in the late fall of 1976, supported with federal grants, but with the larger Mayo Clinic Kasson facility nearby, it closed three years later. Dr. Aquilino stayed on with the Olmsted Medical Group for three years and then left for an academic position in Erie, Pennsylvania. Mayo Clinic's family practice program became an independent department in 1984. Students from the new Mayo Medical School rotated through various departments of the Olmsted Medical Group, but only the Olmsted Medical Group's pediatricians had faculty appointments, and after a time only the pediatrics department hosted students. Second-year students regularly rotated through that department until 2007. Now only a few fourth-year students spend elective time with the Olmsted Medical Center's pediatricians.

* * *

In the spring of 1975, Dr. Ingrid Neel joined the Olmsted Medical Group's pediatric department and established an allergy practice which eventually consumed most of her office time. She was born in Estonia, which was invaded by the Soviet Union about the time of her birth. The Soviets deported many Estonians, especially the educated and the leaders, and moved in Russians. In 1944, Dr. Neel's father, a high school science teacher and principal and active in the underground, was captured and sent to the Gulag. Her mother and three children escaped and came to New Jersey after World War II as displaced persons. In medical school at the State University of New York Downstate in Brooklyn, she met Bryan Neel, whose father was a surgeon in Albert Lea. Her father was released after 20 years in captivity, just in time for their wedding in 1964. Dr. Neel completed her pediatrics and allergy residencies at Mayo Clinic, where her husband joined the ear, nose, and throat department.[126]

As inflation and growth increased the value of the Olmsted Medical Group's accounts receivable, it became more expensive for new physicians to buy shares in the corporation. This problem was an impediment to recruiting and retention. Dr. Wente proposed a change in which the receivables would no longer be a factor in the stock price, lowering the buy-in price by more than 75%. The existing shareholders were compensated by deferred compensation on retirement. This was really the first step toward becoming a non-profit organization. The younger doctors realized that we would in time be buying the investment of the first generation, but no one would be buying ours from us. This disparity was a factor in some physicians leaving the Olmsted Medical Group, but in each case there were other reasons as well. The majority of the physicians felt that the change was for the long-term good of the organization and, therefore, for the individuals as well. Starting in 1976, each new physician was expected to become a shareholder by buying 20 shares of stock at the end of each of five years for a maximum of 100 shares.

In 1976, the Olmsted Medical Group adopted another new practice which is common today. Sister Joyce Hassett, a local Franciscan nun and nurse practitioner, joined the Olmsted Medical Group and began to make regular rounds on all its nursing home patients. By seeing the patients between their physician visits, she improved their care and reduced their time in the hospital, which was good for the cost of healthcare as well as for the

---

[126] Neel, I.V., Interview, Nov. 27, 2007.

patients' well being (but not so good for the hospital's finances). Few clinics employed nurse practitioners then, and most treated them the same as other nurses. In Minnesota, the St. Louis Park Clinic was the only other group to permit them to work at a higher professional level.

The Olmsted Medical Group's keen interest in practicing high-quality medicine led to a visit by Dr. Leonard Rubin, a quality expert from California. He came to the Olmsted Medical Group in February 1976 to review its systems and had several useful suggestions that were adopted. One was implementing a system to ensure that each physician received and signed all laboratory, EKG, X-ray, and other reports before they could be filed in the patient's chart. Before charts were returned to files, they had to be checked by the audit desk to ensure that the reports had been signed. This system required some new expenses, but more importantly, it reduced the likelihood of the kind of tragedy that can lead to malpractice suits. This system has been superseded in recent years by digital signatures in the electronic medical record, a much more efficient process. The willingness of the Olmsted Medical Group to incur additional expenses solely for the improvement of medical care is a characteristic that lives on today.

The Olmsted Medical Group had small numbers of physicians in each department, and departures of physicians had major consequences for the remaining physicians in the department. For example, when two obstetricians, Dr. Bob Rivan and Dr. Sally Schneider, left the Olmsted Medical Group in 1976, Drs. Kaese and Doyle were seriously overworked until Dr. Maggie Fontana, the wife of a Mayo Clinic thoracic disease physician, began practicing office gynecology at the Olmsted Medical Group, and Dr. Rosalina Abboud, who had been practicing in Zumbrota and whose husband is an endocrinologist at Mayo Clinic, also joined the obstetrics department. The Olmsted Medical Group realized that continued growth would help to mitigate some of these disruptions and that recruiting of new physicians to enlarge the size of clinical departments was crucial to the success of the Olmsted Medical Group.

A major addition on July 1, 1976, was Dr. Gary Oftedahl, a native of Westby, Wisconsin, and graduate of the University of Wisconsin and its medical school. He completed an internal medicine residency at the Gundersen Clinic and came to Rochester while his wife did a pediatrics residency at the Mayo Clinic. When she finished her program, she returned to La Crosse, but he stayed at the Olmsted Medical Group for more than 25 years. Dr. Oftedahl had hardly arrived when he and I were drafted to join the board of the Mayo Clinic-backed, newly forming Professional Services Quality Council (PRSO) of Minnesota. Our mission was to "keep an eye on what they are up to." We kept a close eye: Within four years, I was its president and Dr. Oftedahl chaired the major committee. This launched both of us on long careers in leading medical- and healthcare-related organizations.

Although there were many changes, challenges, and some missed opportunities during these years, the Olmsted Medical Group continued to develop as a high-quality medical facility by adding physicians, changing the organizational structure to facilitate ownership by all the physicians, upgrading its information systems, establishing branch clinics, expanding the role of the medical director, and improving the quality and safety of medical care. The Olmsted Medical Group formed a patient education department and hired a nurse to do hospital discharge planning, now a required element of hospital operation. The hospital discontinued tobacco sales at last. Economic changes, inflation, price controls, and increasingly intrusive government programs buffeted both the Olmsted Medical Group and the hospital. Olmsted Medical Group physicians became active participants in efforts to improve the healthcare system and began to take on more important roles in leadership at regional and state levels.

Chapter 6
Troubled Times at the Olmsted Community Hospital

When Mr. Linville retired as administrator of the Olmsted Community Hospital, he was succeeded by Gerald D. Truscott, an assistant administrator at St. Marys Hospital in Duluth. Mr. Truscott quickly found some major problems. When he opened his desk on his first day on the job, January 2, 1975, he found a number of unpaid and unrecorded bills. Worse, the Olmsted Community Hospital was dated and showing its age—most patient rooms had no toilets, the building was in poor repair, and a walk around it revealed a ridge of crumbled brick and mortar on the ground along the circumference. The building needed a major upgrade, but funds were not available. A quick change to a more modern hospital management style was needed.

Mr. Truscott found that the county had not allowed depreciation to be funded. Normally, the value of a building or equipment is depreciated, and an equivalent amount of money is placed in an account to provide for its eventual replacement. In addition, bad debts had never been written off, and there was no system for collecting overdue bills. The hospital also lacked a rational salary system: Some employees were markedly overpaid while other salaries were below market. The previous summer, the Hotel, Hospital, Restaurant and Tavern Employees Union Local 21 had signed a contract to represent a group of hospital employees, mainly because of pay issues. Mr. Truscott recommended expanding and remodeling the hospital and moving the Olmsted County Health Department to its first floor. This would move all the patient care to the second floor and solve the problem of patients having to pass through the main lobby to use the public elevator. He planned to address the inadequacies and disparities in employee pay, to establish a line of communication with the Olmsted Medical Group, and to recommend adding a physician and an accountant to the hospital board.[127] Mr. Truscott contracted with Rochester Methodist Hospital to provide pharmacy services, and the hospital passed its reaccreditation survey in July.[128] But after only eight months on the job and before accomplishing much of what he planned, Mr. Truscott left at the end of August 1975, returning to Duluth to become the assistant administrator of the Duluth Clinic.

---

[127] Olmsted Medical Group Board Minutes, June 9, 1975.
[128] Olmsted Community Hospital Staff Executive Committee Minutes, June 19 and July 17, 1975.

Under public pressure from the hospital medical staff and with Mr. Truscott's recommendation, the county board appointed Dr. Richard Christiana, a family practitioner at the Olmsted Medical Group who had recently served as president of the hospital medical staff, to the Olmsted Community Hospital Board of Directors. The long-overdue appointment provided the Olmsted Medical Group with direct access to the hospital and county boards. When the Olmsted Medical Group's physicians were only a small part of the hospital staff, the separation may have been appropriate, but by this time, the fortunes of the Olmsted Medical Group and the Olmsted Community Hospital had long been closely intertwined, and they needed more open communication between their boards.

Following Mr. Truscott's departure, Jim Cannady, the hospital's assistant administrator, was appointed interim hospital administrator until James E. Brunsgaard took the position on October 1, 1975. Mr. Cannady had been an orderly when the hospital opened in 1955 and became a licensed practical nurse, a registered nurse, purchasing manager, and then assistant administrator.[129] Mr. Brunsgaard had a master's degree in healthcare administration and was the administrator of the Hastings State Hospital, which was slated for closure.

The hospital needed new automated laboratory equipment and had no funds, so in December, the county board approved a $36,000 loan for the purpose.[130] The hospital finished 1975 with a $120,000 deficit—a figure that would later be revised upward. Mr. Brunsgaard arranged a meeting on January 27, 1976, between the hospital and county boards to discuss the financial problems. Major factors were the push by Medicare and private insurers to treat more patients outside the hospital and efforts to reduce the lengths of stay for those who were hospitalized. Thus, in contrast to the overcrowding in the 1950s and 1960s, bed occupancy was now running 50 to 55%. The boards agreed to form a task force comprising Mr. Brunsgaard, county administrator Richard Devlin, and selected hospital and county board members to recommend actions. In the meantime, Mr. Brunsgaard was to carefully consider whether to fill staff vacancies and to raise room rates, which were below those at other local hospitals.[131]

---

[129] *Rochester Post-Bulletin*, June 26, 1980.
[130] Olmsted County Board Minutes, Dec. 16, 1975.
[131] *Rochester Post-Bulletin*, Jan. 28, 1976.

A newspaper article about this meeting broached the possibility of closing the hospital. Coming out of the blue, this shocked many employees and patients, and became the first of many articles to anger the physicians and employees, who saw the negative publicity as compounding the problem. Mr. Brunsgaard soon wrote a letter to the editor trying to put the possibilities in perspective and stating that the article had overemphasized the possibility of closure.[132] In June, Dr. Hartfield and Mr. Wilkus met with Mayo Clinic's Dr. Hodgson and Mr. Fleming, who stated that the Mayo Clinic would support renovation of the Olmsted Community Hospital.[133] The Olmsted Medical Group's executive committee then met with Mr. Brunsgaard to discuss the financial and political situation.[134]

In September, Mr. Brunsgaard closed the hospital laundry and contracted with Dison's Cleaners and Launderers for linen and laundry service, expecting to save about $20,000 a year. In November, the county board contracted with the Minnesota Hospital Association to perform a study "to assist the hospital advisory committee established [in January], to project future healthcare needs and propose ways of putting the hospital on firmer financial ground." Mr. Brunsgaard bravely added that "… there is no possibility that the hospital will close." The advisory committee decided "There is no question the hospital has a role to play in the community. We just have to define what that role will be."[135]

In January 1977, Paul Ludowese, a St. Marys Hospital administrator, was added to the Olmsted Community Hospital board.[136] The Olmsted Community Hospital also decided to hire a comptroller to assist the administrator with financial issues. Mr. Brunsgaard announced that the hospital's loss for 1976 was $66,200, down significantly from $215,000, the audited figure for the previous year.[137] He emphasized that the hospital had no problems meeting payrolls or paying bills, and was not considering closing its doors.[138]

---

[132] *Rochester Post-Bulletin*, Feb. 6, 1976.

[133] Olmsted Medical Group Executive Committee Minutes, June 11, 1976.

[134] Olmsted Medical Group Board Minutes, June 15, 1976.

[135] *Rochester Post-Bulletin*, Nov. 8, 1976.

[136] Olmsted County Board Minutes, Jan. 18, 1977.

[137] Subsequently it was reported that the hospital had also actually lost $55,401 in 1974, Mr. Linville's last year.

[138] *Rochester Post-Bulletin*, May 13, 1977, p. 7.

In June 1977, the long-awaited Minnesota Hospital Association report about the hospital was released. The *Rochester Post-Bulletin* headline blared, "County Hospital Bankrupt in 1981," adding in small print "if it doesn't resolve its financial problems." The 130-page report proposed two options. The first was for the hospital to reduce its capacity to 52 beds, remodel to make the hospital more attractive, reduce staff, and implement other cost-saving measures to save about $400,000 annually. The second option was to close the hospital building and consolidate it with Methodist or St. Marys as a hospital within a hospital. The report also suggested the possibility of selling the hospital to a for-profit chain. Low occupancy and high nurse staffing ratios were emphasized as problems. The report also stated that the hospital still did not have a true budgeting system or a system for managing accounts receivable. It also mentioned several areas of employee dissatisfaction that were causing low morale.

Reaction to the report was varied. Dr. Fred Banfield, then a Olmsted Medical Group physician and the hospital medical staff president, was quoted in the newspaper article as supporting the remodeling proposal, but called the proposal for a hospital within a hospital "implausible." Dr. Hodgson, a member of the Mayo Clinic Board of Governors and of the task force appointed to study the Olmsted Community Hospital, did not speak for the Mayo Clinic but "saw problems implementing the consolidation idea." In a separate article the same day, Dr. Eugene Mayberry, chairman of the Mayo Clinic Board of Governors, and Howard Winholtz, the Methodist Hospital administrator, expressed strong support for the remodeling option. Dr. Mayberry stated that "the reasons for establishing the Olmsted Community Hospital 22 years ago are as viable as or more so than the original reasons."[139]

But the county board was more skeptical. The *Rochester Post-Bulletin* reported that the consensus of the commissioners was to hold off making a decision about remodeling until they were satisfied that the hospital could keep itself in the black. Commissioner Carol Kamper added that the board should have a clearer idea of the Olmsted Community Hospital's role in the next few years when the Mayo Clinic's proposed community medicine program would be underway and the effects of Methodist Hospital's just-opened obstetrics wing would be known.[140] On June 9, the *Rochester Post-Bulletin* ran an

---

[139] *Rochester Post-Bulletin*, June 7, 1977.
[140] *Rochester Post-Bulletin*, June 8, 1977.

editorial headlined "The Crisis at Community Hospital." The editorial stated that, "It would be a tragedy to let Community Hospital go down the drain. Community is a needed facility, providing a needed service." There followed a flood of letters to the editors, almost all supporting keeping the hospital open.

In the midst of the crisis, Mrs. Bohmbach, the well-respected director of nursing since the opening of the Olmsted Community Hospital in 1955, retired on June 30, 1977. Dessa Preuhs, who had been a nursing administrator at Methodist and director of nursing at Hastings State Hospital while Mr. Brunsgaard was there, replaced her a few weeks later. She had also been involved in nursing education, which was an added qualification. She was well acquainted with nurse staffing standards and quickly corrected the staffing ratios.

The financial crisis led to criticism of Mr. Linville's management of the hospital. Several former hospital board members defended him, pointing out that under the county board's charter to the hospital, no disbursements could be made from the hospital fund for long-range planning and funds could not be accumulated for future goals. They also mentioned the cost of paying off the bonds for the 1968 project.[141] Mr. Linville submitted a six-page report to the county board at its September 27, 1977 meeting, defending his administration, which he felt was being unfairly maligned. In fairness, it should be pointed out that this was the only hospital in the state that was expected to be self-sufficient. The other public hospitals operated with tax subsidies, and the private hospitals like Methodist and St. Marys had charitable contributions. Given the constraints under which it was forced to operate, the Olmsted Community Hospital had done tolerably well for a long time.

Joe Cartney, who was a Medicare auditor, became the hospital comptroller on August 1 and quickly discovered several problems. He found that the budgeting process was deficient and he instituted a contemporary budget process; he also obtained an IBM System 3 computer for accounting and management of accounts receivable. The Olmsted Community Hospital had never submitted its rates to the state's Rate Review Commission for approval, so the first submission was for a 20% increase. The commission approved that increase and a smaller double-digit increase the next year.[142]

---

[141] *Rochester Post-Bulletin*, Aug. 2, 1977.
[142] Cartney, J.C., Interview, Nov. 24, 2007.

On August 8, 1977, the county board announced a possible plan to move the health department from its building to the second floor of the Olmsted Community Hospital and to expand the obstetrics wing to create more hospital rooms. The county welfare department, which was leasing the Olmsted Medical Group's Third Avenue building as well as other space, would move into the health department building. By 1980, the county would have $1.2 million in its building fund, and it would save the rent for the welfare department under the proposal. The county board engaged Architectural Design Group to study the feasibility of the hospital expansion. The county attorney noted that expansion of the hospital, even without bonds, would require a referendum or special legislation.[143] County health department officials immediately objected to the plan, fearing that the health department would lose its identity.[144] In November, the architect reported that the proposed plan was feasible. The health department would fit into the second-floor space and could have a separate entrance. A new second floor over the obstetrics wing would replace 40 beds with 25 new ones for a total capacity of 56 beds. The cost was estimated at $1.3 million to $1.6 million, whereas it would cost about $1.9 million to remodel the existing hospital and construct a building for county offices.[145] The proposal was modified to provide 62 beds and was discussed at the December 7 county board meeting.

There was no consensus about how to pay for the plan, but there were several suggestions as the controversy played out in the newspaper: The doctors should pay for it; there should be a community fund drive; or county offices could share space in the soon-to-be-vacated Central Junior High School building. Commissioner Rosemary Ahmann again raised the idea of a hospital within a hospital at Rochester Methodist Hospital.[146] The Olmsted Medical Group repeated its opposition to that.[147] The Olmsted Medical Group felt that a hospital within a hospital would lead to its rapid demise because if its patients had to be hospitalized downtown with the attendant inconveniences, many would just go to Mayo Clinic, St. Marys, or Methodist in the first place. The Olmsted Medical Group felt that Mayo Clinic did not want Olmsted Medical Group physicians at Methodist any more than the Olmsted Medical Group wanted to be there, and a Mayo Clinic spokesman said that the cost of

[143] Olmsted County Board Minutes, Aug. 8, 1977; *Rochester Post-Bulletin*, Aug. 9, 1977.
[144] *Rochester Post-Bulletin*, Aug. 10, 1977, Sep. 28, 1977.
[145] *Rochester Post-Bulletin*, Nov. 23, 1977.
[146] *Rochester Post-Bulletin*, Dec. 7, 1977.
[147] *Rochester Post-Bulletin*, Dec. 13, 1977.

remodeling or adding on to do that would be prohibitive anyway. Throughout the latter part of 1977, there had been multiple meetings between the Olmsted Medical Group, Mayo Clinic, and Olmsted Community Hospital board members to discuss the various options. They also considered the possibilities that Mayo Clinic and the Olmsted Medical Group would cover the hospital's deficits and that Mayo Clinic obstetrics or family medicine departments or medical students would use the hospital. They did not expect the county board to provide ongoing support for the hospital but continued to push the board to renovate the hospital and to do it properly.[148] The year ended with letters to the editor both for and against the proposal with the county board expected to make a decision in January 1978.[149]

The battle of letters to the editor in the newspaper continued into the new year. The *Rochester Post-Bulletin* urged action in a January 10, 1978 editorial. In weighing the pros and cons, the editorial prophetically mentioned that moving the welfare department into the health department building could be a problem because that building was in a flood plain. On January 31, the county board decided to proceed with the renovation plan if a certificate of need were granted as expected and if voters approved a $625,000 general obligation bond issue to supplement the available $975,000.[150] The Olmsted Medical Group board of directors met the next day and recommended the following: (1) opposition to combining the public health center with the Olmsted Community Hospital; (2) encouragement of a management contract with either Methodist or St. Marys hospital; and (3) creation of a financial advisory committee that included administrators from the Olmsted Medical Group, Mayo Clinic, and Methodist and St. Marys hospitals for ongoing review of the Olmsted Community Hospital's finances. The Olmsted Medical Group board planned meetings the following day with Sandy Keith, the Olmsted Community Hospital board chairman, Mr. Fleming and Dr. Hodgson from Mayo Clinic and Mr. Devlin, the county administrator.[151]

The *Rochester Post Bulletin* responded to the county plan with an editorial February 2, panning the "triple play" and pushing for simply remodeling the hospital with the available funds. On February 8, the *Rochester Post-Bulletin*

---

[148] Olmsted Medical Group Board Minutes, Oct. 11, Nov. 8, and Dec. 13, 1977.
[149] *Rochester Post-Bulletin*, Dec. 14 and 24, 1977.
[150] *Rochester Post-Bulletin*, Feb. 1, 1978.
[151] Olmsted Medical Group Board Minutes, Feb. 1, 1978.

again pushed for action and abandonment of the "tri-part shuffling plan." The state law governing county hospitals was vague and ambiguous, but to be safe, the editorial writer favored seeking special legislation to allow the county to finance the project since the Legislature was in session and could act relatively quickly. Alternatively, the editorial suggested, a referendum could be held in May along with the school board elections.

On February 14, the *Rochester Post-Bulletin* reported on the Olmsted Medical Group's efforts to encourage the county board to move ahead with the hospital project with available funds and without a referendum. Two days later, Drs. Wente and Banfield and Mr. Wilkus met with Mr. Keith and Art Birdseye, a hospital board member, to work on a strategy to convince the county board to renovate the hospital adequately. On February 22, a group of civic leaders attended the county board meeting and urged the pursuit of special legislation to get the hospital project moving. The board voted three to two against that proposal, but agreed to hold a special meeting two days later. Commissioner Ahmann said she supported seeking special legislation the next year (1979). County board chairman Gerald Tiedeman wrote an opinion piece for the *Rochester Post-Bulletin* supporting the move of the health department to the hospital in keeping with the original vision in 1947.[152]

At its special meeting, the county board agreed to pursue special legislation rather than a referendum, and Sen. Nancy Brataas and Rep. Kenneth Zubay agreed to sponsor it. The board still planned on the "tri-part shuffle," moving the hospital medical-surgical unit, the health department, and the welfare department. Although it was late in the legislative schedule, Senator Brataas managed to get the bill passed unanimously on March 6.[153] Two days later, the bill was approved by a House committee, but an amendment was inserted by Commissioner Ahmann's friend, Rep. Linda Berglin[154], requiring a referendum if 5% of county voters petitioned for one.[155] The House passed the amended bill on March 11, the Senate agreed to that version two days later, and Governor Perpich signed it on March 22, 1978.[156]

---

[152] *Rochester Post-Bulletin*, Feb. 22, 1978.
[153] *Rochester Post-Bulletin*, Mar. 6, 1978.
[154] Now Senator Linda Berglin.
[155] *Rochester Post-Bulletin*, Mar. 8, 1978.
[156] *Rochester Post-Bulletin*, Mar. 11, 13, and 23, 1978.

Throughout this contentious period, there continued a barrage of letters to the editor on both sides of the hospital renovation issue. The most prolific writer in favor of simply closing the hospital was Glenn Meyers of Byron, an IBM department head. He immediately started a petition drive to force a referendum, which was ultimately successful. On June 20, the county board scheduled the referendum for September 12, 1978, in conjunction with the state primary election. Meanwhile, on April 19, the Southeastern Minnesota Health Systems Agency endorsed the hospital project and recommended it to the commissioner of health for a certificate of need. While all this transpired, Mr. Brunsgaard faced increasing pressure from the hospital board to move faster on the recommendations in the Minnesota Hospital Association report. He resigned effective July 31,[157] and Jim Cannaday was again appointed acting administrator.[158]

The battle over the fate of the hospital was interrupted by another great flood in 1978. Following six inches of rain on July 1, it began raining again on Wednesday, July 5. Through the night, seven more inches of rain fell over the entire South Zumbro River watershed as well as those of the creeks feeding into it in Rochester. By early the next morning, the water was flowing into and over Rochester. A friend whose home was flooded awakened Dr. Wente in the early morning hours. Dr. Wente called Mr. Wilkus, and they set out to check on the Olmsted Medical Group building. The streets being flooded, a deputy sheriff took them in by boat. They found water up to the front door, which they sandbagged, and cold clear water coming up through the floor of the medical records department in the basement. They called their children as well as some doctors and employees, and working together, they saved all of the records threatened by the rising water. Mr. Wilkus managed to procure several pumps to dry out the area.

The regular Thursday morning hospital staff education meeting was scheduled for seven o'clock that morning, so I awoke at six with the radio reporting that the bridges southwest of the city were flooded and closed, followed by a report about the closure of Twelfth Street. By the time I left home, Broadway and Fourth Street were closed. I crossed on Seventh Street with water up to the roadway; it closed five minutes later. The city was soon completely cut in half, with the Olmsted Community Hospital the

---

[157] *Rochester Post-Bulletin*, June 17, 1978.
[158] *Rochester Post-Bulletin*, July 24, 1978.

only medical facility east of the river except for the state hospital. Tragedy struck at the National Health Enterprises nursing home[159] next to Bear Creek when a short circuit caused the elevator to default to the basement, drowning two patients and two staff members. All the other patients were evacuated, the sicker ones to the Olmsted Community Hospital and the rest to the state hospital. The hospital had plenty of doctors present for the staff meeting with nowhere else to go. There was a shortage of most other staff, though, except the nurses who had been on duty before the flood. Mr. Brunsgaard made sandwiches for everyone in the kitchen. By late afternoon, the routes across town were open and things settled down, but the extra guests from the nursing home stayed for over a week.

As the flood subsided, the county board appeared to have scrapped the triple shuffle and planned a $1.3 million renovation of the hospital alone.[160] In mid-June, when it seemed that the petition drive would succeed, a referendum steering committee had been formed, headed by Sandy Keith and including leaders from the Olmsted Medical Group and the Mayo Clinic and its hospitals. Brochures promoting passage of the referendum were included in the August Olmsted Medical Group billing statements and were handed out in the offices.

The steering committee obtained a booth at the county fair in August to be staffed by a doctor and hospital board or auxiliary member. The booth stood between two main aisles and next to a cross aisle, so it was a prime location. I happened to be paired with Sandy Keith, who worked one aisle while I worked the other. No one wanted to talk to me. They all wanted to talk with Mr. Keith, who was and is Rochester's all-time most popular political figure.[161] I talked with two or three people about the referendum, but mostly just watched the master at work. It was an amazing experience. He knew everybody, their kids, and their dogs. The efforts seemed to be working because most of the letters to the editor remained favorable.

The county commissioners decided they wanted more direct involvement in the hospital, and on August 29, they voted to expand the hospital board

---

[159] Now Golden Living Center Rochester East.

[160] *Rochester Post-Bulletin*, July 20, 1978.

[161] Now retired, he is a former state senator, lieutenant governor, and chief justice of the Minnesota Supreme Court.

by adding two commissioners, Douglas Krueger of Rochester and Richard Chase of Chatfield. The county board considered an offer by Methodist Hospital to manage the Olmsted Community Hospital, but declined the proposal because it would have cost more than an administrator's salary.[162] The referendum steering committee held town meetings to promote the referendum.[163] The *Rochester Post-Bulletin* ran supportive editorials on both September 5 and September 6. Its news stories on September 7 covered both sides of the debate extensively. Jane Belau, a prominent community leader, helped with public relations and hosted a viewer call-in program on local public access television the day before the vote. In the end, the referendum on September 12 carried by more than a three-to-one margin.

On November 7, after interviewing three finalists, John W. Allen was appointed hospital administrator, starting January 1, 1979.[164] Mr. Allen had been an assistant administrator at Mary Greeley Hospital in Ames, Iowa, and administered the 112-bed Story County Hospital in nearby Nevada, Iowa. He had what the Olmsted Community Hospital needed—experience in a large hospital along with direct management of a smaller one. Mr. Allen had a master's degree in industrial relations and had done graduate work in hospital administration. On December 5, the county board chose Hammel, Green and Abrahamson as architects for the hospital renovation.

Although overshadowed by the financial and political troubles, other things had been going on at the hospital. In 1975, a utilization review plan was adopted to comply with new federal regulations. Some physicians had questioned the need for routine admission tests for syphilis, which hospitals had required for decades. A review of records showed that there had been only one true positive syphilis test in 1,290 patients and that one was already known to be permanently positive; thus, all the tests had changed nothing. The staff voted to discontinue the requirement.

Mr. Allen's first day as administrator of the Olmsted Community Hospital was January 1, 1979, the same day I became president of the medical staff. I was on call that holiday weekend, and when I went in to make rounds on New Year's morning, I was surprised to see John already at his desk on the

---

[162] *Rochester Post-Bulletin*, Oct. 17, 1978.
[163] *Rochester Post-Bulletin*, Aug. 31, Sep. 1, 1978.
[164] *Rochester Post-Bulletin*, Nov. 4 and 7, 1978.

holiday. He asked me to join him after rounds, and we had a long visit getting to know each other and exchanging ideas about various issues involving the hospital. His two major tasks were to get the hospital's finances in order and to complete the building project. He immediately instituted a more active collection policy for overdue bills, which brought in an additional $177,000 in revenue in the first six months.[165] A new control system for supplies was instituted, saving an estimated $100,000 per year. Noreen Davis moved from Forest City, Iowa, to become the director of nursing.[166] There was an acute shortage of nurses then, and the bad publicity about the Olmsted Community Hospital hampered recruiting. A group of senior nursing students was hired as nursing technicians, and they proved to be very useful.

To improve employee morale, Mr. Allen decided to have a hospital picnic at Quarry Hill Park. Employees, board members, and doctors all attended. Craig Betcher manned the grill, and the picnic was a great success. It was also illegal or at least contrary to county policy, we soon learned—one of the consequences associated with county ownership of the hospital. The county considered the picnic to be an unauthorized employee benefit, because none of the other county employees had a picnic. To avoid possible legal entanglements, the medical staff and auxiliary quickly paid for the event and sponsored the hospital picnics for several years afterward.

The hospital building project took much of Mr. Allen's attention. In contrast to the two previous hospital building projects in 1955 and 1968, the medical staff had considerable input for this one. The staff leadership was included in meetings with the architects, and Dr. Oftedahl and I designed the new intensive care unit. In March 1979, the county board accepted the renovation plan, which addressed nearly all the issues the staff had raised.[167] At the June staff meeting, Mr. Allen reported that the project was four weeks behind because of delays by the architects. In August, the problem became clear as estimates came in about 75% over budget.[168] The increased costs required seriously scaling back the renovation, including eliminating a much-needed replacement for the emergency department and the second

---

[165] *Rochester Post-Bulletin*, Nov. 7, 1979.
[166] *Rochester Post-Bulletin*, Jan. 9, 1979.
[167] *Rochester Post-Bulletin*, Mar. 28, 1979.
[168] *Rochester Post-Bulletin*, Sep. 5, 1979.

elevator to end patients' trips through the front lobby. The losses were a disappointment, but there was hope of revisiting those projects in a few years if the finances improved. Contracts for the renovation were awarded on October 16. Alvin Benike was the general contractor, with Sanitary Plumbing and Heating doing the mechanicals.

The hospital auxiliary hosted an open house on October 28 to show the plans to the public. A brochure highlighted the improvements, which included the intensive care unit; 11 new private rooms, 10 with private bathrooms; new heating, ventilation, and air-conditioning systems; and new beds and modern furnishings for all the patient rooms in the original part of the hospital.

Since there was to be no addition, a ground-breaking was not possible. Instead a "wall-breaking" took place on November 19, 1979. The new intensive care unit was to be in the vacant original labor and delivery area at the end of the south hall on the second floor. We decided to ceremonially break through a wall in that area with a sledgehammer. The walls were constructed of glazed tile to about shoulder level, with plaster above. The softer plaster seemed to be an easier target, as the tile was very hard. The first swing of the sledge hammer was met with a hand-tingling "boing" as the hammer rebounded briskly. We saw that under the plaster the wall was built of hard unglazed tile. After multiple swings by several macho participants, we eventually punched a hole through the wall and declared victory.[169]

One valuable boost for the project was that the hospital hired a "clerk of the works," a retired construction superintendent who represented the hospital and proved invaluable in working out the many problems and details involved in reconstruction. Aside from an eight-week delay due to slow delivery of steel doorframes and the headwall units[170] (the wall-mounted power and utility units at the head of patient beds), the construction went smoothly. The *Rochester Post-Bulletin* published updates, and the project was essentially completed by the end of 1980.[171] It was completely finished in March 1981, with a surplus of $120,000, which was added to the new depreciation fund.

---

[169] *Rochester Post-Bulletin*, Nov. 20, 1979, p. 11.
[170] Olmsted Community Hospital Staff Minutes, Mar. 6, 1980.
[171] *Rochester Post-Bulletin*, Mar. 18, June 26, Oct. 30, 1980.

Meanwhile, the Olmsted Community Hospital Foundation was established.[172] Mr. Allen was able to report to the county board that the hospital was well on its way to a second straight profitable year.[173] The hospital gained favorable notice about its birthing rooms, which permitted labor and delivery in the same room and were the first of their kind in the area.[174]

Noreen Davis, the nursing director, announced in December that nursing students from the College of St. Theresa would begin clinical rotations at the hospital. Olmsted Medical Center no longer has St. Theresa students, but it currently has nursing students at the hospital from Rochester Community and Technical College, Riverland Community College, Winona State, and the RCTC Registered Nurse Refresher program.

An exciting event occurred on August 24, 1981. As I was driving east on Center Street to pick up my son from soccer practice at one of the fields near the hospital, I saw a cloud of black smoke. As I got closer, I thought, "That could be at the hospital." Sure enough, there were fire trucks and police cars, and several of our patients were sitting on the lawn. The soccer team's goalie, who was facing the hospital, had noticed someone in the hospital garage starting a fire. He yelled to his teammates who were facing him. My son Rick and the Abboud's son Mark ran into the emergency room to sound the alarm. The emergency department personnel didn't believe the two boys, though, and had to see for themselves before calling the fire department. Meanwhile, a coach pulled a tractor out of the garage while another coach and the rest of the team ran after the perpetrator, who was no match for a well-conditioned soccer team and was easily captured a few blocks away. They brought him back to the police, who let him slip away, only to be captured by the team again. He was an escapee from the state hospital, where the firefighters were already extinguishing two small fires he had started there. Fortunately, the damage was not severe, the hospital proper was in no danger, and the patients were soon back in their beds. The story and pictures made the front page of the *Rochester Post-Bulletin*.

As 1982 progressed, the Olmsted Community Hospital was anticipating with apprehension the coming change in Medicare payment. Instead of

---

Rochester Post-Bulletin, Oct. 30, 1980.
[173] Ibid.
[174] *Rochester Post-Bulletin*, Mar. 18, Aug. 19, 1980.

being paid based on its costs, the hospital would be paid a fixed amount for each patient admission based on the patient's major diagnosis, a system called Diagnosis Related Groups (DRGs). DRGs provided an incentive for hospitals to discharge patients quickly because they were paid the same amount regardless of how long the patients stayed or how many services they used. The hospital did a market study, which Mr. Allen shared with the Olmsted Medical Group board, confirming the findings of a study the Olmsted Medical Group had commissioned in 1980. The study revealed that a majority of Olmsted Medical Group patients used the emergency department at St. Marys rather than the Olmsted Community Hospital even for minor emergencies. On a positive note, the hospital's Community BirthCenter received favorable notice for the installation of birthing beds, a further advance that enabled delivery of the infant not only with the mother lying on her back but also in a sitting position, which some considered more natural.[175]

When the state hospital closed in 1981, Olmsted County acquired the property and used a portion to house various service agencies including the Zumbro Valley Mental Health Center, a drug detoxification unit, and a community corrections facility. This presented an opportunity for the hospital to expand its services, and in the spring of 1982, Mr. Allen arranged for the hospital kitchen to provide meals to these agencies, as well as laboratory, pharmacy, and housekeeping services, making more productive use of hospital assets whose costs were largely fixed.[176] Due to publicity about dangerous objects being put into Halloween treats, the hospital offered to X-ray them. The radiology department found one pin in a bag of M&Ms that year.[177]

The main challenge at the hospital in 1983 was dealing with the effects of the change to payment by DRGs, not only by Medicare but also by some of the private payers, who often followed Medicare's lead on reimbursement issues. In addition, Medicare was requiring many procedures to be performed on an outpatient basis. These two policies led to a sharp drop in hospital censuses nationwide, and small hospitals were especially hard-hit. Many

---

[175] *Post-Bulletin*, Aug. 4, 1982. The *Post Bulletin* dropped *Rochester* from its masthead as of May 10, 1982.
[176] *Post-Bulletin*, June 11, 1982.
[177] *Post-Bulletin*, Nov. 1, 1982.

hospitals closed or merged during this period. At the Olmsted Community Hospital, 17 surgical operations were performed on an outpatient basis in 1982; just two years later, there were 310.[178] Surgeons began to perform procedures in the office that had previously been performed in the hospital, and physicians treated medical patients who would previously have been hospitalized on an outpatient basis. Obstetrical deliveries increased, but more mothers were discharged on the second day. Hospitals also had to invest in new computer systems to deal with the changes in the payment system.

With fewer patient admissions and an increasing financial burden, the Olmsted Community Hospital continued efforts to increase its visibility, and as part of this plan, the hospital adopted a logo in April 1983. In addition, the *Post-Bulletin* reported favorably on four new programs: two early development classes, an emergency dental call system, and a fitness event. The physical therapy department started a parent and child early development class.[179] While the obstetrics department had offered classes for expectant parents for several years, it began a series for expectant older siblings as well.[180] In addition, an emergency dental call system was launched in November, led by oral surgeon Dr. Robert Gores, the senior member of the dental staff.[181] The hospital, along with the Olmsted Medical Group and the Rochester Track Club, sponsored a new running event in the fall, "Stride for Fitness," which continued annually for 25 years.

Although there was much turbulence and controversy during this period in the history of the Olmsted Community Hospital, lasting progress was achieved in several areas. The hospital acquired a new administrator and implemented modern management methods, improving the balance sheet. A battle over remodeling and upgrading the hospital reached to the State Legislature with a successful outcome, the referendum to approve the construction passed handily, and the hospital survived a threat of closure. Collaboration between the hospital and the Olmsted Medical Group was strengthened after the county board appointed a Olmsted Medical Group physician to the hospital board for the first time and the medical staff

---

[178] Olmsted Community Hospital Operating Room Log Books.
[179] *Post-Bulletin*, Nov. 8, 1983.
[180] *Post-Bulletin*, Nov. 18, 1983.
[181] *Post-Bulletin*, Nov. 24, 1983.

provided input for the hospital renovation. The hospital became the first in the area to launch the new concept of birthing rooms, a service that remains very popular at the hospital today.

In October 1983, John Allen announced that he would be leaving in December for a position with a large hospital-nursing home system in Vermont. He was highly praised for turning around the Olmsted Community Hospital while carrying out a major renovation.[182] Many people associated with the hospital considered him the best administrator that the hospital had during its independent existence. Mr. Allen's departure led again to some discussion of selling the hospital to a for-profit company or outsourcing the administration. The Olmsted Medical Group strongly supported hiring a new administrator and keeping the hospital independent. The county board agreed and Lynn Olson, the assistant administrator, took over in the interim. There was never again talk of closing the hospital.

---

[182] *Post-Bulletin*, Oct. 4, 1983.

Chapter 7
Troubled Times at the Olmsted Medical Group

At the same time that the Olmsted Community Hospital was struggling for its existence, the Olmsted Medical Group was encountering a turbulent period, too. The effort to keep the hospital alive and properly renovated was a dominant issue for the Olmsted Medical Group, since the closure of its only hospital would have dealt it a fatal blow as well. The Olmsted Medical Group felt that the hospital-within-a-hospital concept at Methodist would have been just as deadly, perhaps only a bit more slowly. The inconvenient downtown location and perceived relegation to second-class status for Olmsted Medical Group physicians would have resulted in a loss of specialists. A remnant of primary care physicians with only an office practice might have persisted for a time, but probably would have eventually closed. Once the decision was made to proceed with the hospital renovation, the Olmsted Medical Group was deeply involved in promoting passage of the referendum and in the renovation planning. The Olmsted Medical Group would then turn its attention to troubles of its own.

Dr. Wente planned to retire from the board and as president of the Olmsted Medical Group at the February 6, 1978 annual shareholders meeting—at the height of the hospital crisis. All agreed that this was not the time, and the meeting was adjourned to the evening of March 6, the day the special bill regarding the hospital renovation passed the Legislature. A few weeks earlier, Dr. Wente had asked me to be a candidate to replace him on the board and said he expected Dr. Burich to become president. I had only been with the Olmsted Medical Group three and a half years and thought it was premature, maybe even a bit presumptuous, for me to run for the board. Dr. Fred Banfield was elected to replace Dr. Wente on the board, but Dr. Burich, who was three years older than Dr. Wente, was not looking for more work and declined the presidency. Others were also reluctant, and Dr. John Brodhun was elected. He had had no formal management experience or training, but pitched in to do his part. Some of the younger doctors had been grumbling that Dr. Wente was too autocratic, and they wanted leadership that was more democratic. This fit Dr. Brodhun's natural style, so he seemed a good choice as the Olmsted Medical Group's president.

When Dr. Wente stepped down, he said that he would stay away from management and just be a practicing physician. Most of the doctors thought,

"Yeah, sure, Hal." But, as always, he was true to his word. Subsequent retiring presidents of the Olmsted Medical Group have followed Dr. Wente's example and have supported their successors from the background.

Long-term planning sessions were held with the physicians in the fall. The majority of the doctors preferred that the Olmsted Medical Group stay small and focus on primary care. They were afraid that adding specialists would provoke the Mayo Clinic and were concerned that, because of its size, Mayo Clinic could seriously damage the Olmsted Medical Group, even accidentally. Some of us, though, thought that the Olmsted Medical Group should be the kind of multispecialty group that it would be if Mayo Clinic were 50 or 70 miles away, within easy reach but not next door. This argument persisted for several years before the Olmsted Medical Group finally agreed that the addition of specialists was necessary to provide the kind of medical care that its patients needed and to remain financially stable.

The HMO issue gained momentum during 1978, consuming a lot of the Olmsted Medical Group's energy. There were four separate efforts to establish an HMO in the Rochester area. Treading cautiously, the Mayo Clinic created a fact-finding committee to study the issue. By January 1979, the Mayo Clinic had completed a feasibility study, and by May, it was proceeding with the planning phase for an HMO.[183] Blue Cross and Blue Shield of Minnesota had recently launched HMO Minnesota, which was active only in St. Paul and Duluth, and its president visited the Olmsted Medical Group to discuss expansion of the program into Southeast Minnesota.[184] Several clinics in Southeast Minnesota, including the Olmsted Medical Group, with Mayo Clinic as an observer, began looking at the feasibility of starting an HMO; they referred to it as the Southeast Minnesota HMO Consortium. In September, they met for presentations by potential management companies, including HMO Minnesota, and in December, they contracted for a feasibility study by the same consultant Mayo Clinic had used.

The most controversial effort was the Southeast Minnesota HMO, mainly sponsored by local labor unions, and with Mr. Wilkus, Mr. Fleming from

---

[183] Olmsted Medical Group Board Minutes, Jan. 9; Executive Committee Minutes, May 16, 1979.
[184] Olmsted Medical Group Executive Committee Minutes, Apr. 26; Board Minutes, May 9, June 13, 1978.

Mayo Clinic, and a few hospital administrators included on the board of directors. It applied through the regional Health Systems Agency (HSA) for a federal grant for start-up costs. The Olmsted Medical Group informed the HMO that it would not agree to a capitated contract with them.[185] A few days later, the HMO board of directors ousted Wilkus, Fleming, and Nicholas Spring from Methodist from its board, citing conflict of interest, even though the conflict had been discussed before their appointments.[186] John Allen, the Olmsted Community Hospital administrator, resigned from the board a few days later.[187] On May 7, 1980, the HSA rejected the Southeast Minnesota HMO's grant request because of missing or misleading information.[188] In addition, Mayo Clinic announced that it was dropping its HMO plans.[189] The HSA again disapproved the Southeast Minnesota HMO grant on May 21. But following intervention by Vice President Walter Mondale, the Department of Health, Education, and Welfare in Washington approved a $198,050 planning grant.[190]

In the midst of all this, Mayo Clinic announced the results of another study that showed that Olmsted County residents were hospitalized 30% less often than the national average and that their hospital stays were 40% shorter, again questioning the need for HMOs.[191] In the end, the Southeast Minnesota HMO effort failed. The clinics' HMO Consortium ultimately fell apart in 1981 when none of the clinics except the Olmsted Medical Group was willing to fund it. The clinics agreed to work individually with HMO Minnesota, but the HMO issue again became dormant for a few years.

The other federal initiative, the Southeast Minnesota Health Systems Agency, caused a stir in 1979. Rochester Methodist Hospital planned to expand its obstetrical unit by nine beds and applied to the Agency for a certificate of need, which was endorsed on August 22, 1979. Meanwhile, the Agency had been working on a regional plan including obstetrics. At a closed meeting on August 16, it approved a plan to tier the hospitals, with Methodist the only hospital permitted to manage high-risk pregnancies. This plan would limit the practices

[185] Olmsted Medical Group Board Minutes, Nov. 13, Dec. 11, 1979.
[186] *Rochester Post-Bulletin*, Dec. 21, 1979.
[187] *Rochester Post-Bulletin*, Dec. 26, 1979.
[188] *Rochester Post-Bulletin*, May 8, 1980.
[189] *Red Wing Republican Eagle*, May, 17, 1980
[190] *Rochester Post-Bulletin*, Sep. 24, 1980.
[191] *Rochester Post-Bulletin*, Sep. 17, 1979.

of the obstetricians at Olmsted Community Hospital and the hospitals in Red Wing, Winona, Austin, and Albert Lea. The limitations on their practices would likely result in a loss of obstetricians at those five hospitals and, in fact, it impaired the Olmsted Medical Group's ability to recruit at a time when there was a desperate need for another obstetrician. The administrators of those hospitals objected to the tier plan, and there was quite a furor, especially in Red Wing, with accusations of violation of the open meeting law. The final plan allowed all the hospitals to continue their existing practices.[192, 193]

At the Olmsted Medical Group in the summer of 1979, Dr. Linda Butterfield joined Dr. Mary Pougiales in the eye department, planning to stay for just one year while her husband, Joe, finished a residency at Mayo Clinic. That "one year" ended in 2008 with her retirement. Like Dr. Ingrid Neel, Dr. Butterfield was not a native Midwesterner. She was born in China, where her father became chief of staff of the nationalist army. He was killed in the shelling of Quemoy in 1958, and Linda and her mother moved to Chicago when Linda was 10. She graduated from the University of Illinois and the University of Chicago School of Medicine, and completed an ophthalmology residency at Yale University.

Dr. James Doyle, Dr. Wente's first partner, retired and moved to Arizona. Dr. Doyle had been on the board of Blue Cross and Blue Shield of Minnesota, and I was elected to succeed him. Serving on this board was a major event in my education, because I learned how a major business and board were run. I met many physician, hospital, and business leaders from around the state, attended national meetings with speakers on medical and business topics, and had many networking opportunities. The knowledge I gained was very important when I became the Olmsted Medical Group president in 1984, and it emphasized the need for our leaders to become educated in management and organizational skills. I have often referred to this experience as my MBA (real MBAs may laugh, but let them).[194]

Dr. Burich decided to retire from the Olmsted Medical Group board of directors in February 1980. I seemed to be the logical choice to succeed him

---

[192] *Rochester Post-Bulletin*, Aug. 2, Oct. 9, 17, Nov. 30, 1979.

[193] *Red Wing Republican Eagle*, Oct. 4, 5, 1979.

[194] The last chairman under whom I served as vice chairman was Gary Stern, the president of the Federal Reserve Bank of Minneapolis. He has sent me their monthly and quarterly publications ever since, which have been a great education in economics.

and was elected unanimously. There were also discussions about succession plans for the Olmsted Medical Group administrator, Mr. Wilkus, and there was a proposal to hire another assistant administrator, preferably someone who could be groomed to succeed Mr. Wilkus when he retired. Larry Thomforde, a Rochester native and graduate of the University of Minnesota, was hired for that position in June. Mr. Wilkus had also suggested getting an administrative intern from one of the new masters programs in the area.[195] There was interest in doing a marketing study to see what the Olmsted Medical Group was doing right or wrong and where there were opportunities to offer new or better services. In his activities with the American Academy of Medical Directors, Dr. Hartfield had met Dr. Eric Berkowitz, a young professor at the University of Minnesota School of Business[196], who taught marketing for the academy. He agreed to do the study, and an intern was hired to assist him. The intern, Thomas Holets, was a Rochester native who grew up in Byron and at the time had finished three years at Concordia College in Morehead.

The study results were reported to the Olmsted Medical Group board in November 1980. A startling finding was that one-third of respondents were not familiar with the Olmsted Medical Group, including 60% of those who weren't the Olmsted Medical Group's patients. Even the Olmsted Medical Group's patients weren't very familiar with its services or hours, and they were even less familiar with the Olmsted Community Hospital. Clearly, the Olmsted Medical Group and the hospital had not been doing an adequate job of marketing and branding. A number of attitudinal areas were examined, including the importance of having one doctor, follow-up procedures, and scheduling. The study found that the Olmsted Medical Group's greatest strength compared to the Mayo Clinic was ease of parking. Dr. Berkowitz made a number of suggestions to improve the Olmsted Medical Group's visibility, and six committees were formed to explore implementation.

By the summer of 1980, the need for marketing was all the more apparent. Patient visits at the Olmsted Medical Group dropped by 5,140 from the first half of 1979. The cause of the large decrease wasn't clear. The problems at the hospital may have been a factor, but patient visits to doctors were down nationally due to the credit crunch as the Federal Reserve System

---

[195] Olmsted Medical Group Executive Committee Minutes, July 26, 1978.
[196] For some years now, Professor of Marketing at the University of Massachusetts at Amherst, and a nationally recognized expert in healthcare marketing.

moved to stop the rampant inflation. In addition, the Mayo Clinic opened a family medicine department in its new Baldwin building, which may have drawn some of the Olmsted Medical Group's patients.[197] While the Olmsted Medical Group had put its retirement fund on the line to build a modest facility, in contrast a major donor gave Mayo Clinic $5 million to fund a program in direct competition to the Olmsted Medical Group. Like the Olmsted Community Hospital, the Olmsted Medical Group didn't have a level playing field either. By November 1980, visits were down by 7,774; collections were $120,000 below budget, and expenses were $100,000 over budget. The shareholder dividend was canceled.[198]

But two new opportunities to improve the Olmsted Medical Group's financial condition arose, one involving insurance exams and the other a new branch clinic. A Mayo Clinic fellow approached the Olmsted Medical Group with a proposition to sell it a large part-time business he had developed performing exams for insurance companies. He had created a very efficient system, which was important to insurance agents who wanted to get the policies sold and in effect as quickly as possible. Because he planned to leave the Rochester area, the fellow offered to sell the business and teach the Olmsted Medical Group's staff the system for a very reasonable price.[199] The Olmsted Medical Group purchased the business, marking the beginning of a successful occupational medicine department. The second opportunity occurred when a group of citizens in Elgin, where Dr. Ellis had retired in 1978, formed a corporation to build a clinic and asked the Olmsted Medical Group to staff it. Mayo Clinic had closed a clinic it had acquired in nearby Plainview, so the area was underserved and could qualify for a Health Service Corps doctor. This was an attractive offer, and the Olmsted Medical Group accepted it.

As 1981 opened, the Olmsted Medical Group looking at long-range staffing needs and the main clinic building's capacity. The Olmsted Medical Group thought it would need four more family practitioners, two internists, a pediatrician, a surgeon, and an orthopedist. The building would accommodate five more doctors, but was designed to expand by two floors. Another opportunity was the pending closure of the state hospital, which would leave a gap in psychiatric care that the Olmsted Medical Group might be able to fill.

---

[197] Olmsted Medical Group Board Minutes, July 14, 1980.
[198] Olmsted Medical Group Board Minutes, Nov. 11, 1980.
[199] Olmsted Medical Group Executive Committee Minutes, Dec. 24, 1980.

The Profit-Sharing Trust had been unable to rent the Third Avenue buildings after the welfare department moved out. After entertaining several offers, the buildings were sold to Donald Monson for $300,000 early in 1981. Remembering Harry Harwick's advice to secure all the land the Olmsted Medical Group could, Dr. Wente opposed the sale and predicted that "… some day we'll buy it back for four times the price."[200] But he was outvoted by Dr. Burich and Mr. Wilkus, the other trustees. The trustees were also becoming more optimistic about getting an exemption from the U.S. Department of Labor to continue owning the Olmsted Medical Group's building because the Everett Clinic in Washington state had been granted an exemption in a nearly identical situation.

The Olmsted Medical Group board decided to hire Mayo Clinic residents to relieve the overworked family practitioners of weekend emergency room call, although they still provided backup. Dr. Nancy Grubbs decided to start an internal medicine residency at Mayo Clinic and planned to return to the Olmsted Medical Group. She later decided to stay at Mayo Clinic, to our great disappointment, thinking that she would probably just resume her family medicine practice if she returned to the Olmsted Medical Group.

The Olmsted Medical Group added another specialty in September 1981, when Dr. Ken Ubben became its first dermatologist. A native of Rockwell, Iowa, he did premedical and medical education at the University of Iowa and a residency at the University of Minnesota. He also trained at the University of Wisconsin with Dr. Frederic Mohs, learning his eponymous technique of skin cancer surgery. Another acquisition was a large sailfish that Frank Sander had caught off Marathon, Florida, which his wife would not allow him to display in their house. The fish hung on the wall of the Olmsted Medical Group's back stairs for several years. After being retired, it starred in the lead role of our production of Dr. Suess' "You're Only Old Once." The fish now resides in the maintenance department of the Rochester Southeast Clinic.

Establishing new branch clinics was a major initiative for the Olmsted Medical Group, and it held meetings with the Elgin community group and with Dr. Jeff Morgan, who along with his wife, Dr. Jeanne Mohler, was finishing a family practice residency in Battle Creek, Michigan. Dr. Morgan, a Health Service

[200] Olmsted Medical Center purchased the property in January 2008 for less than twice the 1981 sale price.

Corps physician, was hired to staff the new Elgin clinic, and Dr. Mohler would work in the Olmsted Medical Group's main clinic, both beginning in July. The Elgin building cost the city more than the estimated cost—and more than the available funds. The Olmsted Medical Group made a generous prepayment of five years' rent, relieving the community association of its financial bind. Meanwhile Tom Berg, a grocer in Stewartville, approached the Olmsted Medical Group about the possibility of opening a clinic in that community in the shopping center he was developing. Dr. Risser, the town's only doctor, was approaching 70, and there was no other physician in the town of nearly 3,000 residents. The Olmsted Medical Group had been interested in having a branch clinic in Stewartville for some time, but didn't want to offend Dr. Risser. After several discussions with Mr. Berg and the Olmsted Medical Group, Dr. Risser accepted a proposal for a two-doctor clinic in Mr. Berg's development. Dr. Risser's independent practice could occupy one side of the clinic for as long as he wanted to work, and the Olmsted Medical Group would staff the other side and provide lab and X-ray services for him.

Dr. Craig Thauwald started up the Olmsted Medical Group's Stewartville clinic at the beginning of 1983 and has led it ever since. He grew up in Preston where his family ran the funeral home. After medical school and residency at the University of Minnesota, he spent a couple of years helping or filling in for small-town physicians in the area while he decided what he wanted to do for the rest of this life. I had first encountered Dr. Thauwald when he was helping Dr. Roland Matson in Spring Valley about a year earlier, was impressed with him, and was excited to have him join our growing practice.

The Olmsted Medical Group marked its entry into psychological services in 1982. Following the dour marketing report from Dr. Berkowitz, the Olmsted Medical Group was looking for assistance in public relations. At the same time, some of the Olmsted Medical Group's primary care physicians thought it would be useful and convenient for their patients to have a psychologist on site. The Olmsted Medical Group hired Dennis Gannon, a psychologist at the Zumbro Valley Mental Health Center, to work half-time in public relations and half time in psychology. He started on August 2, became overwhelmed with psychology patients very quickly, and had little time for his public relations job. The provision of psychological services proved to be a vital component of the Olmsted Medical Group, and the department grew rapidly, eventually to 13 psychologists and psychiatrists.

The Olmsted Medical Group board held a retreat in September 1982 to begin long-range planning to bring it to 40 physicians, which some experts were saying was the optimal size for medical groups. Mr. Tomforde, the assistant administrator, had left, and his position was open. Dr. Brodhun and I recommended hiring Tom Holets, who had been employed to assist Dr. Berkowitz with the marketing study and was in a master's program at the University of Iowa College of Medicine. He was scheduled to complete the program in May 1983. However, there was a possibility that he could do his residency with the Olmsted Medical Group starting in December 1982, and Mr. Wilkus managed to arrange that. The board thought that Mr. Holets could get five or six years of experience under Mr. Wilkus, and then fill the administrator position when Mr. Wilkus retired. Mr. Holets's first assignment was to oversee the installation and implementation of a new computer system. When the Olmsted Medical Group started computerized appointment scheduling, the receptionists were terrified, but they quickly found the system to be very efficient and would not part with it. Subsequently the Olmsted Medical Group developed an experienced information technology department to smooth the transitions occurring with each addition of computer and software systems.

There were other changes in the Olmsted Medical Group staff that year. Dr. Frank Sander, a general surgeon, retired in May 1982 and moved to Las Vegas. He had become quite a proficient blackjack card counter and planned to make some extra retirement income there, which he did for a while until the casinos caught on to him. Dr. Clayton Bennett, a family physician, retired in June.[201] Dr. Harry Burich, the Olmsted Medical Group's senior surgeon, had expected to retire before Dr. Sander since he was older, and he was not eager to take on any more work in Dr. Sander's absence. He decided to reduce his schedule to half-time on July 1 and to not take call except to cover my afternoon off and the week I was at the American College of Surgeons meeting in October. He planned to retire completely at the end of 1982.

The Olmsted Medical Group energetically embarked on recruiting another surgeon. Fortunately, Dr. Charles Branch, whose father was a successful surgeon in Peoria, Illinois, visited in November and agreed to join in late January 1983. A graduate of Northwestern University Medical School, he completed a residency in Santa Barbara, California, where one of his teachers was a surgeon who had been one of my chiefs in Chicago. Dr. Branch spent

---

[201] Dr. Bennett died Nov. 8, 2008.

six months in London with one of England's top surgeons, and then a year in a regional hospital in Swansea, Wales. Dr. Branch became the ideal partner, always willing to work his schedule around mine, which made my leadership activities at the Olmsted Medical Group and elsewhere possible.

The Olmsted Medical Group was affected by a severe recession in 1982 as the Federal Reserve continued to squeeze inflation out of the financial system. Patient visits and charges continued to increase, but collections were down. Costs were increasing, and the Olmsted Medical Group had made several significant investments and commitments, including a pledge of $50,000 for the expansion of the Mayo Civic Center, more than it could really afford. There was increasing worry about finances. It was thought that improvement with public and community relations could help, and in December 1982, a community advisory committee was assembled to assist.

The Olmsted Medical Group continued to work on marketing, sometimes coordinating with the Olmsted Community Hospital, trying to make its services better known and exploring opportunities to meet the needs of the community. Like the hospital, the Olmsted Medical Group adopted a logo and a consistent color scheme for printed materials. It also published a patient information brochure, which included pictures of all the doctors and their specialties. Several areas with a potential for growth were evaluated, including addiction treatment. Dr. Garber had developed expertise in the treatment of alcoholism and other chemical dependencies. He and Mr. Gannon met with Greg Gahnstrom, a local chemical dependency counselor, to suggest the possibility of starting a new type of treatment program. The program would combine a brief period of inpatient treatment with a longer period of intense outpatient therapy. Mr. Gannon also suggested starting an employee assistance program, initially to serve our own employees, but that could be offered later to other employers. A third idea was an employee wellness program, again for Olmsted Medical Group's use at first, but to be marketed later.[202] In August 1983, the Olmsted Medical Group contracted with Mr. Gahnstrom to conduct a feasibility study for a chemical dependency unit. The plan and its risks were explained to shareholders, who approved the proposal. By year's end, the program had a business plan, a budget, and the name of Daybreak; and Mr. Wilkus was negotiating for space on the former state hospital campus. He said the unit would be "the economic salvation of the Olmsted Medical Group."

---

[202] Olmsted Medical Group Board Minutes, June 8, 1983.

In keeping with the general desire for more participatory governance, the Olmsted Medical Group board recommended a change in the bylaws to reduce the board term from five to three years and to provide a limit of two consecutive terms except for that of the president, who could serve three. The board also discussed the Olmsted Medical Group's salary system to address some concerns of the newer doctors. Although physician salary systems may seem to be a pedantic issue, in reality such systems are a crucial component of recruiting and retaining high-quality physicians. A stable, equitable, and evenly applied system complements the primary motivating factors for physicians, which are the style of practice, delivering high-quality care, relating to colleagues, and the communities where they live. Dr. Oftedahl, who had joined the board in 1982, suggested that the Olmsted Medical Group look at the Gundersen Clinic's salary system. The Gundersen administrator, Ed Carlsson, visited and explained the system. This plan was discussed at the September 1983 staff meeting, and the Olmsted Medical Group adopted a modified version based on a survey of midsize group practices in the Midwest. With minor adjustments, this system survived over 20 years—possibly a record for physician salary systems.

By May 1983, there had still been no action by the U.S. Department of Labor on the Olmsted Medical Group's request for an exemption from the requirement that the Profit-Sharing Trust sell its main building. The Olmsted Medical Group's attorney recommended that the trust sell the building to a physician partnership, which would return us to the situation that had existed 13 years previously. The partnership would have tax advantages for the partners, converting rent into capital gains. Aside from some correspondence, little progress was made on this through the rest of the year.

Despite an auspicious beginning, 1983 was probably the worst year of the Olmsted Medical Group's existence. The major challenge of the year was a severe decline in the Olmsted Medical Group's financial position. The effects of the recent recession were still being felt in the reduced collections, and Medicare's DRG system reduced payments to physicians as well as hospitals. Medicare paid doctors on hospital service a certain amount per day, and as lengths of stay shortened, doctors earned less. They were still doing the same amount of work, or even more, because the patients in the hospital were sicker on average than before and required more care. The doctors at the clinic were also working harder and earning less. Patients who would formerly have been treated in the hospital were now outpatients, consuming more of the doctors' time and effort at lower fees. Medical Assistance now paid only about 40% of actual charges, which was even less than Medicare. Several new physicians had been added in a short time so not all of them had full schedules yet, but they still had to be paid. Costs increased even more because of increases in capital spending in the past year. By May 1983, collections were slowing again, and the deficit was $80,000 and getting worse. The second quarter ended with a $90,000 deficit, mostly because of a sharp decline in the collection ratio and fewer visits per doctor in the newly enlarged family medicine department.

Mr. Wilkus presented a list of possible responses to cut costs, extend office hours, and monitor charges. By the end of September, the deficit was down to less than $5,000. Accounts receivable, though, were still $350,000 more than a year earlier. The board held meetings with each of the departments to explain the situation and solicit ideas for improvement. The schedule for the medical staff meeting was changed so that it would occur shortly after the board met, improving the communication flow. The Accreditation Association for Ambulatory Health Care carried out its triennial reaccreditation survey in late August, and the surveyors seemed well satisfied with the Olmsted Medical Group's quality of care. However, when the surveyors presented their report a few months later, the Olmsted Medical Group was shocked to find that it had been accredited for only one year. Accreditation officials explained that it was because they expected us to be out of business before then.

By December, things were improving, but worries remained. Collections were better, and there was an $80,000 profit for the year. But the Olmsted Medical Group still could not afford dividends or profit-sharing contributions. Mr. Wilkus warned that with the new salary plan starting in January, we would be starting 1984 in a dangerous financial position. Dr. Brodhun had been a steady leader for six years through difficult periods of inflation and recession as well as increased competition and regulation, but he had not been eager to be president and decided that he would not stand for re-election in February.

Despite the turbulence of these years, the Olmsted Medical Group added specialties and upgraded equipment. Branch clinics started in Stewartville and Elgin, and psychological services were added. At the end of 1983, the we had 30 physicians, 13 of them in family practice; net revenues of $5.1 million; and $66,109 in net worth. Like the Olmsted Community Hospital, the Olmsted Medical Group had survived a brush with extinction. We were still in business, though, and there was hope that the worst was over.

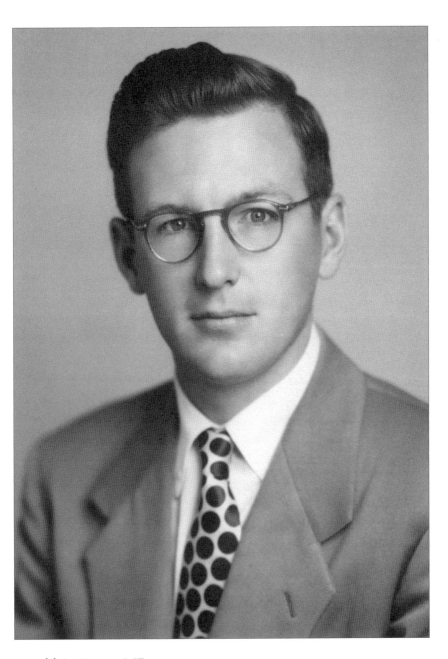

Harold A. Wente, MD
c. 1955, Courtesy of Harold A. Wente, MD

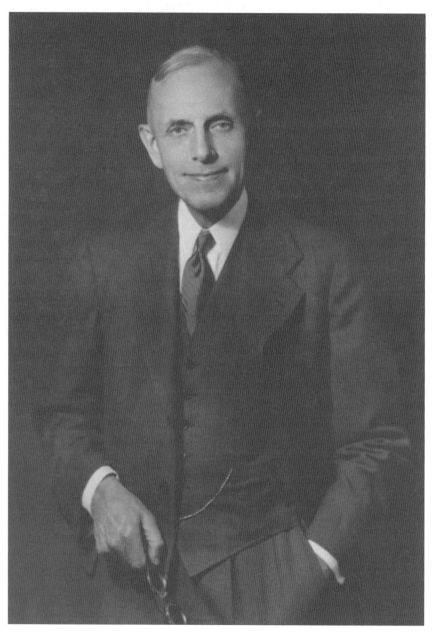

William F. Braasch, MD
1954, By permission of Mayo Historical Unit, Mayo Clinic, Rochester, Minnesota

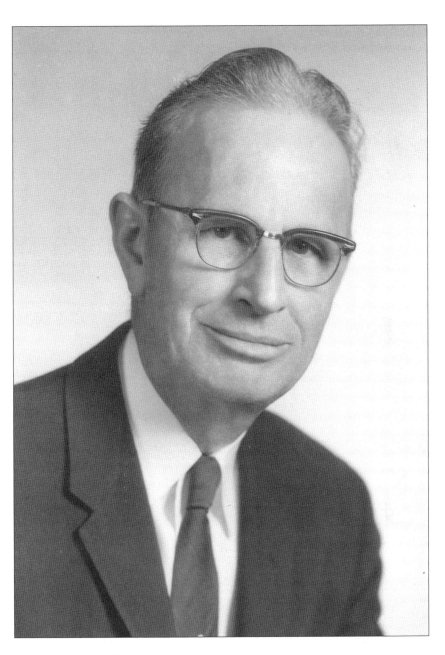

Cedric M. Linville
c. 1955, Courtesy of OMC Hospital Auxiliary

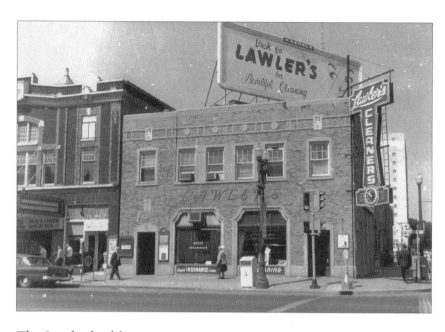

The Lawler building
c. 1957, Courtesy of History Center of Olmsted County

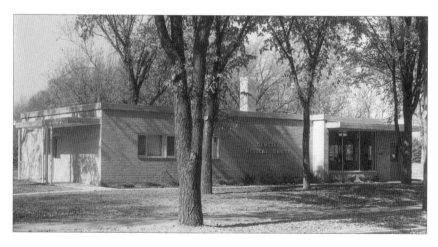

Olmsted Medical Group – Third Avenue building
1953, Courtesy of Harold A. Wente, MD

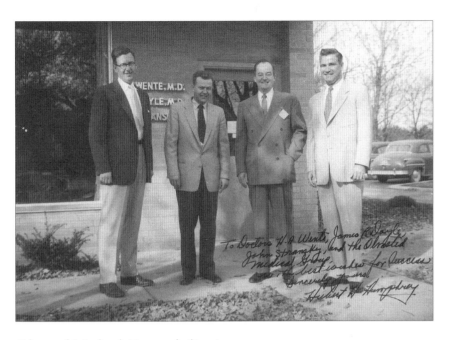

Olmsted Medical Group dedication
(L to R:) Harold A. Wente, MD, John J. Stransky, MD,
        Senator Hubert H. Humphrey, and James R. Doyle, MD
August 1953, Courtesy of Harold A. Wente, MD

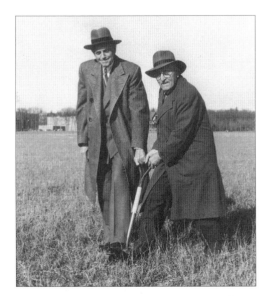

Olmsted Community
Hospital ground breaking
(L to R:)
William F. Braasch, MD,
O. P. Giese
April 13, 1954, Courtesy of
OMC Hospital Auxiliary

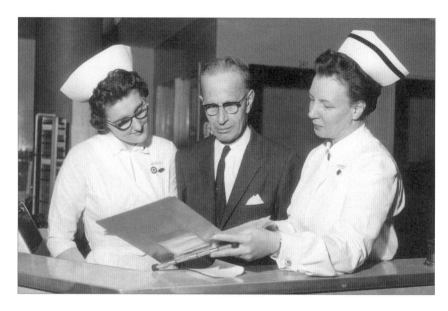

(L to R:) Evelyn Heil, Surgical Nurse; Cedric Linville,
        Hospital Administrator; and Julia Marchant (Bohmbach),
        Director of Nursing at second floor nursing station
1955, Courtesy of OMC Hospital Auxiliary

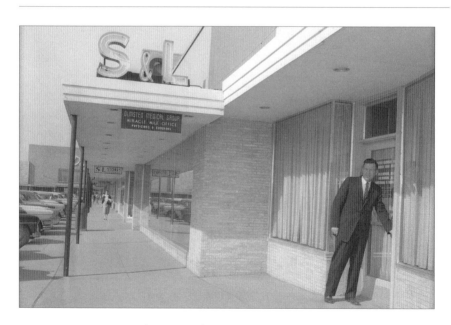

Dr. Wente entering the second Miracle Mile clinic
c. 1957, Courtesy of Post-Bulletin

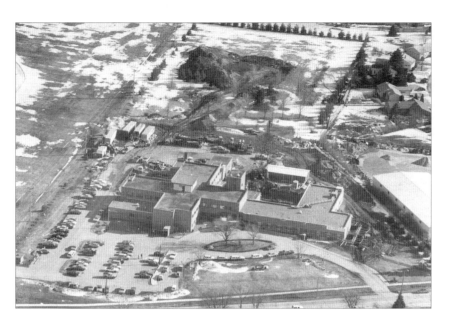

1968 Hospital addition, near completion
Courtesy of Post-Bulletin

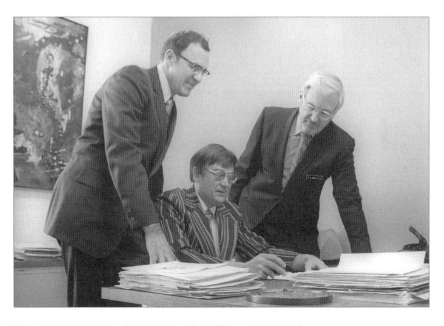

(L to R:) Dale Hawk, MD, Frank Wilkus, OMG Administrator,
        and Harold A. Wente, MD, establishing the St. Charles satellite clinic.
December 1, 1972, Courtesy of Post-Bulletin

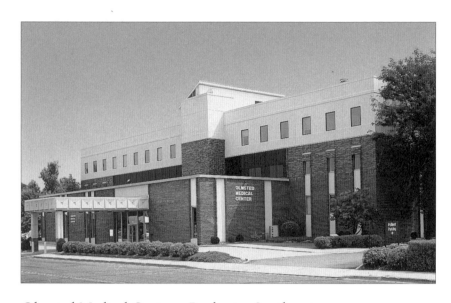

Olmsted Medical Center – Rochester Southeast
c. 2008

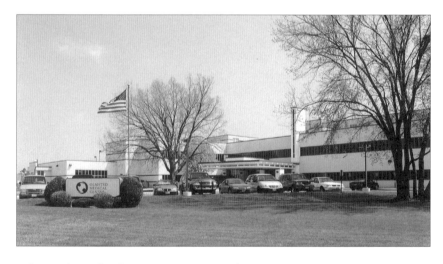

Olmsted Medical Center – Hospital
c. 2008

Part II: Out of the Shadow

Minnesota Medicine:
"Dr. Geier, the Olmsted Medical Group
is rapidly growing, even though it sits in
the shadow of the Mayo Clinic."

Dr. Geier:
"First of all, we are located southeast
of the Mayo Clinic, so we are never in their
shadow. However, early on a winter morning when
the sun hangs low on the southeast horizon ..."

Interview, *Minnesota Medicine* 73:13, 1990.

Chapter 8
Changing of the Guard

At the beginning of 1984, the Olmsted Medical Group was still in a precarious financial position, and there was a strong bias for action throughout the organization. The board was facing a critical decision about choosing a successor to Dr. Brodhun. There was a presumption among many physicians that I would be his successor, but Dr. Oftedahl expressed an interest in the position and both of us were nominated at the February 14 board of directors meeting. The two of us left the room, leaving three board members to decide the issue. After some discussion, including that I was better at business and Dr. Oftedahl was a better people person (both of which were true), I was elected two votes to one, a good ratio but not much of a margin. Dr. Werner Kaese perhaps expressed the sentiments of the Olmsted Medical Group the day after the election: "I don't care what you do, Dick. Just do something. And whatever you do, I'm behind you 100%." At the annual shareholders meeting on February 13, Dr. Malcolm Campbell, the last original board member, had retired from the board, and Dr. Ingrid Neel was elected to replace him.

Immediate action was necessary on several fronts. Aside from shortening the board meetings from an average of five hours to just over three, the first issue was that of physician productivity, which had been a problem almost from the Olmsted Medical Group's beginning. The new productivity-based salary system was being instituted, but the productivity survey showed that nearly all the Olmsted Medical Group's doctors were near the bottom for their specialties by regional standards. The recent period of rapid inflation resulted in an equally rapid increase in costs and fees for medical services. The doctors were uncomfortable with the higher fees and often charged for less time than they actually spent with patients or didn't charge at all for some visits. In addition, most of the physicians valued lifestyle more than maximizing income and saw fewer patients than average. This low productivity resulted in physician incomes that were well below average, which made it hard to recruit specialists and to retain physicians, and contributed to the Olmsted Medical Group's financial problems. I decided on a radical approach to the problem. With the board's approval, I announced to the Olmsted Medical Group physicians that their salaries would be increased by 10% or to the 20th percentile, whichever was greater, and, by the way, we didn't have the money to pay them at these levels. Either we were going to get to work and make a competitive income, or the Olmsted Medical Group would go bankrupt and we could move somewhere else where we could make a living. Having lit the fire, there were double-digit increases in productivity in each of the next three years.

Another urgent matter was that of administrative succession. Tom Holets, the new assistant administrator, was just 25 years old. He had interned at the Olmsted Medical Group in the summer of 1980 after his third year of college. After his internship he earned a master's degree at the University of Iowa and was now working on an MBA at the University of Minnesota. When he started work with the Olmsted Medical Group in December 1982, the plan was that he would gradually take over while Mr. Wilkus phased out over five years or so. But the financial and other problems of the last two years had taken a toll on Mr. Wilkus, and it was apparent that his retirement timetable would accelerate. In December 1983, I had been at a national Blue Shield meeting where one of the speakers was Tom Peters, a co-author of *In Search of Excellence*, a best-selling management book. Tom, Dr. Hartfield, and I started meeting weekly and discussing the book, getting to know each other better, and developing a consistent philosophy and management approach.[203] Despite his young age, I felt that Holets was bright, well educated, and up to the job of administrator. Mr. Wilkus agreed to stay on for a year or two as executive director to provide advice or to help with specific projects. He also suggested that his office be off-site to avoid ambiguity as to who was the administrator, and an office in the Olmsted Medical Group's old Third Avenue building was rented for him.

The ownership of the Ninth Street building by the Profit-Sharing Trust had been made illegal by the Employee Retirement Income Security Act of 1974, but the Olmsted Medical Group had had 10 years to comply. This had been the best investment for the trust, returning 12% a year regardless of the stock market or bond rates. By the time the application for an exemption was denied, the Olmsted Medical Group could not meet the deadline and had to pay a penalty. A new partnership of physicians, Olmsted Medical Properties, was organized to purchase the building, with Dr. Neel, the newest board member, named as managing partner. The process was complicated by the fact that Lutheran Brotherhood owned the

---

[203] One of the points in the book was the importance of developing a "mythology" of the organization, a sense of its history and purpose. Two outgrowths of this are the portraits of past leaders in the Rochester Southeast Clinic's administrative corridor and this book.

land on which the building was situated; but it ultimately provided the financing for the new partnership to buy the building. For several years, the IRS had been forcing down the valuation of the building to reduce the tax-deductible rent that could be charged. Now, however, the U.S. Department of Labor ruled that the valuation of the building should be raised for the purpose of the sale to protect the interests of the beneficiaries of the profit-sharing trust. The partnership's down payment was thus a much smaller portion of the price than they had anticipated, and all of the partners were required to individually pledge their lives and sacred fortunes, such as they were, to Lutheran Brotherhood. When the deal was finally completed in May 1985, the Profit-Sharing Trust had $2.3 million in cash for the trustees, Drs. Wente and Burich, to invest in the stock and bond markets. Because the rent was based on the value of the building and the need to meet the mortgage payments, the properties partnership had to raise the rent sharply for the Olmsted Medical Group, which could ill afford it.

Daybreak, the Olmsted Medical Group's planned chemical dependency treatment center, was progressing, but with a lease to be negotiated and a number of details to be worked out. One delay was due to a requirement that the county advertise for bids on the space the Olmsted Medical Group was going to rent, and when the bidding was held, the Olmsted Medical Group was the only participant. Mr. Holets managed the project, and the center opened on July 2, 1984. The program was an innovative one, combining two weeks of inpatient therapy with four weeks of intensive outpatient treatment. This lowered the cost significantly from the then-standard six weeks of inpatient care only. Unfortunately, the demand for Daybreak's services was less than expected, and collecting payment was difficult. By the end of 1984, the deficit was almost $115,000.

The Olmsted Medical Group's executive committee began to meet regularly with Dr. Gene Mayberry, Mayo Clinic's CEO, and Bob Fleming, its administrator, to keep each other informed of plans and to avoid surprises. They said that Mayo Clinic wasn't planning an HMO and assured us that the Olmsted Medical Group would be included in any alternative healthcare financing arrangement they might consider. Blue Cross and Blue Shield started requiring pre-authorization for hospital admissions in August 1984, then began its Aware Gold program with a 40% discount for physician services, which the Olmsted Medical Group could not afford. Medicare then came out with a program in which it would pay "participating physicians" directly if they would accept Medicare's fee schedule. This fee schedule represented a 45% reduction in the Olmsted Medical Group's usual fees, so the it declined that as well, although it later did become a Medicare participant after Minnesota law was changed to essentially require it.

In September, Dr. Oftedahl and I attended our first American Group Practice Association[204] meeting. As it had for Dr. Wente, this organization became a major source of education for us, as well as a way to meet other group leaders from around the country and discuss mutual issues. We brought back many ideas over the years that could be employed at the Olmsted Medical Group. The current leaders of the Olmsted Medical Center also continue to derive much benefit from attending the meetings.

The annual board retreat was also held in September. The board discussed external relationships—with employers, insurers, competitors, and others. Most of the time was spent considering the mission and corporate culture of the Olmsted Medical Group and the relationship of the organization and individuals to each other. Employee morale was a point of discussion. One issue affecting morale was that there were two small, adjoining employee lounges, one for smokers and one for nonsmokers. The lounges were too small, and smoke filtered into the nonsmokers' area. The division of employees was also not desirable. The board decided to combine both lounges into one smoke-free area. The board also decided to eliminate smoking in all of the Olmsted Medical Group's clinics by January 1, 1985. After the retreat, Mr. Holets discussed the idea with the supervisors, nearly all of whom smoked. They surprisingly suggested that the smoke-free date be moved up to November 1. And so the Olmsted Medical Group became the first smoke-free medical clinic in Minnesota, twenty-three years before the state made it mandatory. The Olmsted Medical Group also started smoking cessation programs, and many employees quit smoking as a result.

Despite ongoing financial difficulties, the Olmsted Medical Group continued its commitment to high-quality medical care and upgraded several pieces of equipment (an ultrasound machine, a mammography unit, and a blood analyzer) and purchased a laser for the eye department. At the end of 1984, the Olmsted Medical Group made a profit-sharing contribution equal to 5% of salaries and entered the new year with some cash on hand.

---

[204] Now the American Medical Group Association.

* * *

The Olmsted Community Hospital also underwent a change of leadership in 1984. Robert Brandt, who had been administrator of the Tomah Memorial Hospital in Tomah, Wisconsin, became the hospital administrator March 12.[205] He had a master's degree in hospital administration from George Washington University and had a record of running building programs at small hospitals. The Olmsted Community Hospital was unusual in being a small hospital whose medical staff consisted almost entirely of members of one multispecialty group. Mr. Brandt had not worked in such a situation before, and miscommunications and misunderstandings developed that made it harder for the de facto system of the hospital and the Olmsted Medical Group to work well together.

Several areas of cooperation between the Olmsted Community Hospital and the Olmsted Medical Group were explored. Lynn Olson, the hospital's assistant administrator, suggested a joint venture with the Olmsted Medical Group to build a clinic in Northwest Rochester; but the Olmsted Medical Group, which was already thinking of that, didn't think that the hospital should be in the clinic business, even as a partner. The Olmsted Medical Group also saw little use for joint ventures with the hospital, because the it could already do about anything a joint venture could do. Mr. Brandt suggested that the Olmsted Medical Group and hospital create a joint pre-admission desk to help patients navigate the rapidly increasing insurance barriers, but the Olmsted Medical Group already was doing that and did not need the hospital's involvement. One area that did look promising for cooperation, though, was physical therapy services. The Olmsted Medical Group had enough space for outpatient physical therapy, but still had not been able to replace Gwen Gunsalas, the long-time therapist, who had retired in 1980. The hospital had a new physical therapy department head and was starting to plan a building program that would temporarily put a lot of hospital space out of commission. Based on expected expenses, sources of patients and the location, an agreement was reached to have hospital therapists deliver outpatient therapy at the Olmsted Medical Group facility, with the hospital and Olmsted Medical Group sharing the costs and profits. There were some concerns about legal issues, but those were resolved and the program took effect in November.

* * *

---

[205] *Post-Bulletin*, Feb. 14, 1984, p. 32.

Mr. Holets took the administrative reins of the Olmsted Medical Group at the start of 1985. The new computer system was becoming fully functional, which helped with financial reporting and industry comparisons, collections, and other functions. Mr. Holets reorganized the collection process; moved the Olmsted Medical Group's banking to Norwest Bank[206] to maximize interest; worked with Ability Building Center, a sheltered workshop, to reduce bulk mailing costs; and brought more modern management techniques to bear. Board members were provided more written materials before board meetings, which required more homework and thought by the members, but made the meetings shorter and more efficient.

To assist my work as Olmsted Medical Group president, I started formal management education in January 1985 with the Physician in Management courses offered by the American Academy of Medical Directors, and continued taking courses in finance, law, marketing, and other areas over the next 10 years. Before the proliferation of master's degree programs for physicians, this was about the only source of formal training for physicians in management and was extremely valuable. I also suggested that the executive team meet with its counterparts in neighboring medical groups, especially the larger ones, to discuss mutual problems and solutions. There were several interesting and helpful meetings of this nature, resulting in new ideas being brought back to the Olmsted Medical Group.

The moribund HMO issue was resurrected early in 1985, and in July, another meeting of the Southeastern Minnesota clinics along with the attorneys for the participating groups was held in Mankato to again consider starting a regional HMO. But the effort fizzled again because most clinics were unwilling to make any investment. Mayo Clinic then told us that it was planning to start an Independent Practice Association type of HMO by the summer of 1986. A further meeting with Ron Anderson and Dr. Dick Tompkins from Mayo Clinic assured the Olmsted Medical Group that it would be included in Mayo Clinic's program, and with little effect on the Olmsted Medical Group's practice or payment. Mr. Holets and Dr. Oftedahl attended the American Group Practice Association meeting in October and heard that HMO penetration was leveling off as standard insurers responded in ways that eroded the competitive advantage of HMOs. Some of the responses by insurers included requiring preauthorization before hospital admissions and second opinions before

---

[206] Now Wells Fargo Bank.

surgery. The former added to costs and the latter proved ineffective because it cost the companies more than it saved. The insurance payers were also pressuring doctors to accept lower fees as "preferred providers."

A new opportunity for the Olmsted Medical Group to expand its reach in the region arose in Pine Island. The town had lost its last physician several years earlier, but had kept the community-owned clinic open on a part-time basis, staffed initially by nurse practitioners and later by Mayo Clinic residents who worked two evenings and Saturday afternoon each week. In February 1985, a group of community leaders met with Mr. Holets to determine whether the Olmsted Medical Group might operate the clinic. Mr. Holets and I visited Pine Island and the clinic, and were impressed with the town's leaders and their vision for its future growth. A marketing study was completed, and in November the Olmsted Medical Group committed to taking over the clinic by July 1986. As it happened, Dr. Allan Clark, who had grown up on a dairy farm near Preston, was interested in working in Pine Island. He worked his way from Rochester Community College to the Mayo Medical School and a family practice residency in Iowa, and had just served for three years in the Air Force. Dr. Clark seemed to have been made for Pine Island's small-town practice. He spent a few weeks in the main clinic and in Stewartville learning the systems, and then opened the new clinic in Pine Island on March 3, 1986.

The Olmsted Medical Group took advantage of another opportunity to expand specialty services with the addition of its first anesthesiologist, Dr. Roxolana Demczuk. Recently married to a Mayo Clinic physician, Dr. Demczuk came from Children's Memorial Hospital in Chicago and had been on the Northwestern faculty. She was more interested in academic medicine than community practice, and the Olmsted Medical Group agreed that, if a position opened at Mayo Clinic, it would release her from her contract.

Daybreak, the Olmsted Medical Group's venture into chemical dependency treatment, continued to struggle. It wasn't attracting enough patients to cover its costs, especially since many of the patients were uninsured and were treated at no charge or reduced charges. There were promises of new state programs that would provide funding for these patients, but the Legislature failed to act on a bill to create them. By the end of 1985, Daybreak lost another $156,000. After considering several options, the Olmsted Medical Group decided to convert it to an outpatient-only program, which would substantially reduce the overhead.

Dr. Hartfield was elected president of the American Academy of Medical Directors, which brought him into national prominence. He was actively recruited by several large organizations, and in October announced that he would be leaving at the end of the year to become senior vice president and corporate staff medical director of Cigna Health Plan and would relocate to Dallas. The board appointed Dr. Oftedahl to succeed him as the Olmsted Medical Group's medical director.

The Olmsted Medical Group ended 1985 with a profit of $368,000 and $108,000 equity despite paying the Daybreak losses. In two years, we had gone from a brush with bankruptcy to our best financial year yet.

* * *

By early 1985, the Olmsted Community Hospital was moving ahead with plans for a building project. After some reluctance, as in 1979, the Olmsted County Health Department agreed to move into the hospital's obstetrical wing and the front part of the original first floor. A new Community BirthCenter would be built directly over the old one. The health department would use the front entrance, and a new entrance for the hospital would be built on the southeast corner of the building. A new emergency department would be built on the northeast corner and a three-story addition would be built on the south side of the building for surgery on the second floor, solving part of the elevator problem. A larger cafeteria and new conference rooms would be on the first floor, with administration and sterile supply in a walkout basement. The still-crumbling brick exterior would receive a stucco-like covering, and there would be a four-bay detached garage.

The physicians were disappointed in having less input in the design phase than they had had in 1979. Mr. Brandt involved a few individual doctors, but the Olmsted Medical Group's leadership was not consulted. I had some involvement with some final details of the operating rooms, and Dr. Jeff Morgan, then the Olmsted Medical Group's emergency department physician, was somewhat more involved in the plans for that department, but most physician input was solicited after the plans were nearly finalized.

There were other contentious issues as well. The joint venture in physical therapy was going well, but access for patients was limited. The Olmsted Medical Group wanted the physical therapists to be available for same-day referrals, and by year end, all-day service was restored. The profits for the first year were greater than expected, and Mr. Brandt wanted to renegotiate retroactively a higher percentage for the hospital. The Olmsted Medical Group's unsuccessful attempts to have its medical director attend hospital staff executive committee meetings also sparked conflict. To top it off, representatives of the Olmsted Medical Group were not invited to the ground breaking ceremony at the hospital on January 8, 1986.

Despite the friction between the hospital and the Olmsted Medical Group, good things were happening at the hospital. The Joint Commission reviewers in May 1985 were very complimentary and said that the Olmsted Community Hospital was in the top 15% of hospitals nationally. At least part of this high-level performance was due to the willingness of the hospital staff to adopt leading-edge technology, for example, the new technique of patient-controlled analgesia (PCA). I had read of the idea for an apparatus developed at the University of Louisville for patients to give their own intravenous pain medication. PCA resulted in more effective narcotic use at lower doses. As soon as the pumps were available in June 1985, the hospital acquired two of them to study with surgical patients. The Olmsted Community Hospital was one of the first hospitals in the country to use PCA, which soon became routine. In July, there were 45 inpatient and 76 outpatient operations, the first time outpatients were a majority.

A new medical records supervisor, Elaine Bassi,[207] arrived in July, and Sue Klenner became the DRG and utilization review coordinator in September. Noreen Davis, the director of nursing, developed a day care program for sick children called Under the Weather, and she created an attractive logo of a duck carrying an umbrella. This program arose from the hospital's effort to keep employees at work rather than stay at home with sick children, and it was opened to the community as well. When necessary, an emergency department physician could see the children and medications could be administered.

* * *

At the beginning of 1986, the Olmsted Medical Group sported an all-new leadership team—a new generation, eager and progressive. The Olmsted Medical Group's finances had improved, the administration was strengthened,

---

[207] Now Elaine Hettwer, Sue Klenner's administrative assistant.

and the organization was positioned for a major transformation. With the changes in healthcare pushing patient care out of hospitals, hospitals were continuing to close or merge. From 1980 to 1985, there was a 40% drop in hospital days throughout the state, and Olmsted Community Hospital was affected as much as the other hospitals. It seemed imperative that, for the hospital to survive, the Olmsted Medical Group had to provide more patients, but without compromising the conservative practice style. The solution was to resolve the Olmsted Medical Group's dilemma about primary versus specialist care and to grow. At the annual shareholders' meeting on February 24, 1986, I announced that the Olmsted Medical Group would become the dominant provider of healthcare in Southeastern Minnesota.[208] This meeting was a major turning point in the development of the Olmsted Medical Group, establishing a vision and strategy that still drive the Olmsted Medical Center more than 20 years later. In my remarks, I stated that:

"We will increase the breadth of our services by making them more attractive—more convenient, efficient, personal; making them more available—more places, more times; increasing our obstetrical services; working with insurers and employers.

We will increase the depth of our services by adding new specialties; increasing staff in specialties that cannot meet demand; adding new services and skills to existing specialties; making better use of internal referrals—educating patients and staff as to what we have available.

This will require several supporting strategies: improving management capability to handle greater volume and multiple sites; improving physician recruitment, orientation, evaluation, and education; increasing space, equipment and personnel; promoting research and development; increasing market research to learn needs of patients, employers, and insurers; and improving marketing to meet the identified needs."

Aided by better salary offers and a new, enthusiastic medical director, recruiting became more successful. Dr. Bob Nesheim became the Olmsted Medical Group's first psychiatrist in May 1986. Dr. Peter Frechette, who had been in private practice in Springfield, Illinois, started the orthopedics department in July. Three new family practitioners came in July, including a second doctor

---

[208] This was some years before the idea of "Big Hairy Audacious Goals" became popular.

for the Stewartville clinic. Dr. Rob Grill, an ophthalmologist practicing in Ann Arbor, Michigan, visited the eye department in the spring and joined the Olmsted Medical Group in August. Dr. Allan Bakke, a former NASA engineer, became the Olmsted Medical Group's second anesthesiologist after he completed training at Mayo Clinic. Dr. Bakke is famous for winning a landmark Supreme Court case concerning reverse discrimination. Dr. Demczuk, the Olmsted Medical Group's first anesthesiologist, moved to Mayo Clinic, and we were soon recruiting a second anesthesiologist.

There were changes in the administration as well. Dennis Etbauer, the Olmsted Medical Group's laboratory supervisor of six years, earned an MBA degree from Winona State University and was promoted to assistant administrator; his duties included purchasing, staffing, ancillary services, and satellite operations. Joe Canney was promoted to comptroller. He had come to the Olmsted Medical Group from the credit department at the Olmsted Community Hospital in 1956 to become the Olmsted Medical Group's credit manager. He had been promoted to assistant administrator about five years later and had done yeoman's work in that position.

With the Pine Island clinic off to a good start, the Olmsted Medical Group explored other branch clinic opportunities. A market study suggested that this was not yet the time for a branch clinic in rapidly growing Northwest Rochester. In June, Dr. Dale Hawk contacted the Olmsted Medical Group to discuss taking over his St. Charles practice again. He was approaching retirement and his associate, Dr. John Balkins, was not interested in buying him out, but Dr. Hawk wanted to preserve the service for the community. The Olmsted Medical Group closed the deal with Dr. Hawk in August 1986, and the clinic reopened on September 1 with a new sign. In July, a committee from Preston asked the Olmsted Medical Group to consider starting a clinic there. However, Dr. Robert Sauer, who had earlier practiced in the area, was planning to return, and the Olmsted Medical Group did not want to compete with him. In October, discussions began with Dr. Matson and his associate, Dr. Brad Westra, in Spring Valley. Like Dr. Hawk, Dr. Matson was planning to retire soon, and Dr. Westra did not want to buy the practice. A market study showed a high level of enthusiasm for the Olmsted Medical Group in the community, and planning for the new branch clinic was begun. An agreement was reached with Dr. Matson, and the Olmsted Medical Group acquired the practice in November 1987.

With the new doctors in the Olmsted Medical Group's Rochester clinic, there was a space shortage. Mr. Holets and I met with Lutheran Brotherhood and Norwest Bank in June 1986 to explore financing and with three architects in September to discuss expansion of the main building. We retained Harold Westin, the original architect, to design a third floor for the entire building except over the entrance. The radiology department requested that the X-ray film files stored in the basement be moved to the department, but their weight required a stronger floor than those in the existing building. We decided to fill in the southwest corner of the building, between the west and south wings, with a three-story addition. This addition would also provide more room for central supply and a for a larger employee lounge on the lower level. The existing building needed refurbishing, too. The professional staff was informed of the plan, and the doctors received questionnaires to outline their space needs and desires as a starting point. For instance, to see true skin color, the dermatologist wanted north or east light, not the more yellow south or west light, a preference that no one would have known without asking.

New financial strains for the Olmsted Medical Group arose when Blue Cross and Blue Shield of Minnesota (BCBSM) responded to price pressures from the HMOs by launching its Aware Gold plan, but this time it went even further by making acceptance of the program, with its markedly reduced fees, mandatory for all physicians who cared for patients insured by BCBSM. Throughout my tenure on the BCBSM board, I had argued that paying all doctors the same, regardless of their quality and efficiency, made no sense.[209] It punished the efficient and rewarded the inefficient. I kept advocating for what is now called "value pricing." The Olmsted Medical Group simply could not accept the deep discounts the insurance payers demanded. Because Mayo Clinic did not participate with BCBSM, the Olmsted Medical Group's physicians were the main providers for them in the area, which gave us some bargaining strength.

At a Blue Shield meeting in Denver in the spring of 1986, Virgil Hammarstad, a BCBSM senior vice president, and I, leaning against a pillar in the Brown Palace hotel one evening, developed the outlines of what was possibly the first pay-for-performance, or value-based, contract. Mr. Holets negotiated the details, and BCBSM used the contract as a model for a few other groups

---

[209] The Mayo Clinic has been forcefully making this same point in the current national healthcare reform debate.

as well. The agreement included participation in HMO Minnesota; and the Olmsted Medical Group was the first in Southeastern Minnesota to work with it. The Olmsted Medical Group was also the first to sign with the Mayo Health Plan, which was launched on August 11. This plan simply paid fee-for-service, but withheld 10% to cover plan losses. The Olmsted Medical Group never received the 10%, and the Mayo Health Plan eventually closed down.

The Olmsted Medical Group's venture in chemical dependency treatment, Daybreak, would have been better named "Daybroke." Because it was now an outpatient program, it was moved to a smaller space. Also, staffing was decreased and advertising was increased, but to no avail. In December 1986, arrangements were made for aftercare for the patients in the program, and it closed at the end of the year. What was supposed to have been the financial salvation of the Olmsted Medical Group ended up costing about $400,000, for which we were left with 20 coffee mugs with the Daybreak logo. I still keep one of those $20,000 mugs on my desk as a pencil holder and as an anti-hubris talisman. It is amazing that Mr. Holets and I kept our jobs, but everything else was going well for the Olmsted Medical Group and all the shareholders had given the Daybreak project their blessings. The fiasco taught the Olmsted Medical Group two lessons: First, don't let the champions of a new program do the feasibility study, and second, make sure the payers will pay before starting.

The Olmsted Medical Group ended the year with a 7% profit-sharing contribution, retained earnings to cover depreciation, and paid off Daybreak's debts. Revenues were almost $7.5 million, up 17.5% from the year before.

* * *

The Olmsted Community Hospital project was off to a good start, but soon ran into delays. Often the workmen would open up a space to place the planned ducts, pipes, or wires, and they would find something else already there that was not on any previous blueprint. Another empty space would have to be found—and there weren't many of them.

Hospitals nationwide continued to be under financial stress, and cost-cutting was the order of the day. The hospital nurses had the impression that the director of nursing, Noreen Davis, had been hired specifically to cut staff, which is indeed what she proceeded to do. Nursing staff morale plummeted.

The doctors thought that the hospital nurses were good at their jobs but that the hospital departments were not functioning well as coherent units. Administrative processes were structured around the hospital staff rather than around the needs or convenience of patients and doctors. Outpatient surgery, for example, could be scheduled only between 9:00 AM and 4:00 PM weekdays and at least 48 hours in advance.

There were bright spots at the hospital too. In addition to the new "Under the Weather" sick-child program, a home healthcare program was started to replace one closed by the county health department. The kitchen began providing the food for "Meals on Wheels," a service that the hospital continued to provide for more than 24 years. In February 1986, almost 75% of surgeries at the hospital were performed on an outpatient basis. Dr. Branch passed the surgery board examination, and he relieved me as chief of surgery. The hospital picnic that summer, again funded by the hospital staff and auxiliary, was a joint getting-acquainted affair with the health department. The hospital medical staff again passed a resolution for a smoke-free hospital in October. It was implemented the next March except for three designated patient rooms.

***

The hospital board invited me to speak at its retreat in September 1986 about the Olmsted Medical Group's structure, history, and plans, as well as what the Olmsted Medical Group wanted from the hospital, the relationship between the Olmsted Medical Group and the hospital, and what the relationship should be. The structure and history were straightforward. I told them about the Olmsted Medical Group's growth and building plans and how they had been largely dictated by the hospital's needs. While the Olmsted Medical Group expected that its bottom line for 1986 would be reduced by over $200,000 because of that growth, the expansion would pay healthy dividends in future security and stability for both the Olmsted Medical Group and the hospital.

I talked about how the Olmsted Medical Group wanted the hospital to exist and to be stable, and how it believed it that the hospital should provide adequate facilities, equipment, and staff. There had been ongoing improvements in all these areas except the hospital staff, which the Olmsted Medical Group felt had been cut excessively, hurting morale and service. The hospital needed to have a better image and better public acceptance. Market studies had consistently shown the hospital to be less well known and less well regarded than the Olmsted Medical Group, and that was hurting us. The Olmsted Medical Group wanted the hospital to foster an attitude of serving patients, their families, and their doctors, and making systems work for their convenience. Hospital prices should be competitive. The cost of outpatient surgery, for example, was considerably higher than the statewide average. This was also an area of vulnerability for the hospital should insurers refuse to pay those prices. The hospital needed to demonstrate flexibility and the ability to adapt to rapid changes such as in surgery, which had gone from 8% outpatient procedures to 60% almost overnight in 1984.

The Olmsted Medical Group wanted its relationship with the hospital to be friendly and cooperative despite all the stresses both organizations were undergoing, I noted. The Olmsted Medical Group was not interested in starting services that would compete with the hospital such as an ambulatory surgery center. Nor was the Olmsted Medical Group interested in having the hospital hire doctors to compete with it. Finally, the Olmsted Medical Group was not particularly interested in joint ventures with the hospital.

All this was probably more than the board wanted to hear. I tried not to be too negative, and there were, in fact, many positives, especially with the building program and the opportunities for improvement it offered. The underlying problem was that the Olmsted Community Hospital and Olmsted Medical Group were seen by the public as a single system, but in fact were not. They were still two separate systems with different management and different directions. It was about this time that I reached a major turning point in my thinking: *How could the two organizations be combined into one larger, integrated healthcare system under unified governance and management?*

Chapter 9
New Structures

The Olmsted Community Hospital had completed its building project, and the Olmsted Medical Group started one of its own. Then the most important new projects were begun—restructuring both organizations.

The Community BirthCenter opened February 10, 1987, and the hospital board approved making it smoke-free. All the rooms were birthing rooms, and the hospital had a new mother-baby nursing program. The same nurse cared for the baby and mother together, and the baby spent more time with the mother, as she desired.[210] Deliveries jumped almost 30% from 1986 to 1988.

Noreen Davis, the director of nursing, announced in March 1987 that she was leaving for a job in Michigan. As I was walking across the hospital parking lot toward her farewell reception, I ran into Sandy Keith, who was also attending. He asked how things were, and I ventilated a bit. He then asked me, "Why don't you guys just take it [the hospital] over?" I told him that I had been thinking about that, but as much as I would have liked to, I saw two problems at present. First, the hospital business seemed risky at this point; the Olmsted Medical Group had just gone through the Daybreak fiasco, and was leery of taking on a project that would consume a lot of time and energy and that could prove to be very expensive. Second, I thought it would appear that the Olmsted Medical Group was trying to steal the newly renovated hospital and that it would not be politically acceptable. Nevertheless, the idea of a merger was alive and not confined to the Olmsted Medical Group's leaders.

Robert Brandt, the hospital administrator, announced in early April that he would be leaving at the end of May for another job and building project in Burlington, Wisconsin. As with most previous hospital administrators, his relationship with the Olmsted Medical Group was sometimes contentious; but he kept the hospital in good financial shape during a difficult period, and the building project accomplished about everything that was possible at the time. Many of the problems were simply because we were trying to run a de facto combined system with two administrations, two boards, and goals that sometimes differed.

---

[210] *Post-Bulletin*, Feb. 11, 1987.

The health department moved into its new space in the hospital in July 1987, and the hospital's new, much improved emergency department opened that August. Karen Wheelock Brezicka replaced Ms. Davis as director of nursing, and Joe Cartney became the interim hospital administrator. Ms. Brezicka had a background in nursing education and a calm, gentle manner. She was just what the nursing staff needed. Mr. Cartney was easy to work with, and he understood the idea that while the hospital and the Olmsted Medical Group each had their own interests to look out for, they also had a strong interest in each other's well being. Communications and working relationships improved when he began to meet monthly with the Olmsted Medical Group's executive committee and, while we didn't always agree, we were always friends.

Even before the health department moved into its offices in the hospital, the county board had been discussing the possibility of a joint administrator for the hospital and health department to reduce the cost for both. Although the idea of combining the hospital and county health departments under a single management seemed attractive, it diverted attention away from the solution that proved best for the hospital, which was a merger with the Olmsted Medical Group. Dr. Arvid Houglum, the public health officer, who was planning to retire in about two years, opposed the idea of having a joint administrator. He feared that a joint budget would shift resources away from public health to the hospital. In addition, his opinion was that the hospital was unrelated to a public health mission.[211] Dr. Bill Taylor, chairman of the board of health, said, "Now is not the time." But Commissioner Howard "Chub" Stewart told Dr. Taylor that he "should put aside the turf fight and start economizing."[212] The hospital board proceeded with a search for its own administrator, but its first choice withdrew in December 1987, and the board put the process on hold, leaving Mr. Cartney as interim administrator. There the matter sat for more than a year.

The hospital building became smoke-free on January 1, 1988, and the grounds followed in April. Passes for patients to go outside to smoke were banned. During this period, the hospital was having difficulties recruiting nurses, especially for the evening shift. Part of the problem appeared to be a lack of day care for nurses' children, especially in the evening. The hospital obtained a matching grant from the Southeast Minnesota Initiative Fund and

[211] Olmsted County Board of Health Minutes, June 6, 1987.
[212] Olmsted County Board of Health Minutes, June 16, 1987.

started an on-site day care center for employees' children named Over the Rainbow. It was busy from the start, but it was closed in August 1992 because of its expense and lack of use by the target employees. Child Care Resource and Referral started New Beginnings at Evangel United Methodist Church and hired most of the employees. Under the Weather, the hospital's day care program for sick children, was closed at the same time for similar reasons.

* * *

In January 1988, Mr. Holets and I met with Richard Devlin, the county administrator, and Bob Bendzick, the county's finance director, to talk about possible scenarios for a merger of the Olmsted Medical Group and the Olmsted Community Hospital. Initially, the Olmsted Medical Group suggested a nonprofit umbrella corporation with a for-profit subsidiary medical group and nonprofit hospital. There was initial skepticism with this idea, but when Mr. Holets posed the idea of the Olmsted Medical Group's becoming nonprofit also, Mr. Devlin agreed to look into the possibilities. One issue was whether the real estate and bond agreements the county had signed to finance the recent hospital addition and renovation would provide any impediments. In May, Mr. Holets met with Kit Freeman, one of our attorneys, to discuss the possibilities of the Olmsted Medical Group's buying or leasing the hospital. Mr. Freeman discussed the issue with Ray Schmitz, the county attorney, who saw no legal problem, and then with the bond counsel. By October, everyone agreed that there were no insuperable obstacles, and the Olmsted Medical Group's executive committee planned to continue to review the possibilities of some type of combined organization.

The Olmsted Medical Group executive committee met with Mr. Devlin on December 19, 1988, to express its own concerns about having a joint administrator for the hospital and the public health department. Unlike Dr. Houglum, the Olmsted Medical Group was afraid the hospital would be disadvantaged by combining the management of the hospital and the health department, and it expressed interest in an eventual merger of the Olmsted Medical Group with the hospital.[213] The next day, the county board decided

---

[213] Shortly before this, I had talked with Commissioner Howard "Chub" Stewart, who is Dr. Craig Thauwald's father-in-law, about the idea of merging the Olmsted Medical Group and hospital in some way. He responded, "That's just a pipe dream. It will never happen." Now, neighbors and friends, I enjoy reminding him of his prediction.

to hire a joint administrator. But the board ran into a legal obstacle because it lacked the authority to hire the public health officer; and it was necessary to restructure the board of health. On June 13, 1989, Dr. James Kurowski was hired as administrator of both the hospital and the health department, to start July 1. Dr. Kurowski was a graduate of Creighton University School of Medicine and had a master of public health degree from Johns Hopkins University.[214] He was in charge of a group of clinics related to Denver General Hospital in the Denver Department of Health and Hospitals. The fact that he had worked in an integrated healthcare system was a big advantage from the Olmsted Medical Group's standpoint. Although Dr. Kurowski became the administrator for both the Olmsted Community Hospital and the health department, the two organizations kept their separate boards, employees, and budgets. Dr. Kurowski answered to both boards and the county board, with Mr. Devlin as his immediate superior.

* * *

At the same time, the Olmsted Medical Group was dealing with its own structure and a restructure. During the first half of 1987, there were meetings with the doctors and employees to develop and review the plans for a building addition. Financing was arranged with Lutheran Brotherhood to provide the permanent mortgage, with Norwest Bank for the construction loan, and with First Bank for a $1 million line of credit. The property partnership added 14 new partners, and 10 of the existing ones increased their investments to help make the down payment. Each of the partners still had to guarantee the entire loan individually.

A groundbreaking ceremony for the expansion was held July 2. There were two main points in the comments I made at the event. First, while the building was an important facility and its expansion marked a milestone in the Olmsted Medical Group's growth, the people in that building were much more important. It was their years of hard work and dedicated service that built the Olmsted Medical Group. Second, the Olmsted Medical Group's growth and expansion came about not because of a major donation or a government grant or subsidy, but because of the willingness of its doctors to invest in the future of the Olmsted Medical Group. These physicians put at risk their life savings, their retirement plans, and their own homes, because

---

[214] *Post Bulletin*, June 14, 1989, p. 1B.

of their confidence that the Olmsted Medical Group would continue to grow and prosper in the future as it had in the past.

The $1.8 million expansion added 23,000 square feet, increasing the building's size by more than half. It was a fast-track design-and-build contract. By mid-August 1987, the steel work was nearly complete, masonry work was starting, and electrical and mechanical drawings were being completed. By October, the project was ahead of schedule and $100,000 under budget, which allowed for inclusion of a second front elevator and other upgrades. Departments moved into the third floor in June 1988, although a portion was left unfinished for future use.

When the Olmsted Medical Group began its growth and building plans, there was some concern that the increased size of the building might detract from the smaller scale and personal atmosphere that patients enjoyed. We needn't have worried. It was interesting and heartening to hear the patients' reactions, the way they identified with us—how "we're" growing and how "our" building is coming along. They were like sports fans talking about how "we" won the big game when they were in the stands or watching on television a thousand miles away.

Building projects were relatively easy compared to organizational restructuring. Because of several problems that had arisen, the Olmsted Medical Group board was again reviewing the organizational structure, a process that lasted most of the year. An increase in retained earnings was needed to buy more equipment for the increased number of physicians, which increased the corporate taxes. In addition, the value of the partners' stock depended mostly on the Olmsted Medical Group's financial results in a given year rather than on any long-term measure. The 1986 tax reform made the property partnership less tax friendly, and Mr. Holets investigated some alternative structures. The Olmsted Medical Group discussed the possibilities of a foundation model, a beneficiary trust, or simply a stated buy-in/buy-out stock price. Despite the tax change, the partnership was still better than double taxation if the corporation owned the buildings. At the board's strategic planning retreat in September, board members again discussed the idea of combining the Olmsted Medical Group and the hospital under a nonprofit umbrella corporation or even a merger. The board also talked about the possibility of nonprofit status for the Olmsted Medical Group, including the advantages of tax savings and tax-exempt financing and the trade-offs needed to make it possible. At this time, the board decided not to pursue nonprofit status but did establish a fixed stock price.

Another incentive to consider applying for nonprofit status occurred in 1988 when the federal tax rate for professional corporations was raised to 34%, a higher rate than for other corporations. At a meeting of the American Group Practice Association's healthcare economics committee, of which I was a member, the Virginia Mason Clinic in Seattle discussed its recent conversion to nonprofit status and the process they used. A major issue in the conversion was avoiding taxation of the accounts receivable because they would be considered income to the old corporation while the tax-deductible expenses accrued to the new one. The Virginia Mason Clinic had solved the problem by running the two corporations simultaneously for a time. I was excited by this possibility and reported it to Mr. Holets later in the day, but learned that he had already been looking into the possibility on his own. The Duluth Clinic had become nonprofit also, and Stan Salzman, its administrator, had told him about their process and the attorney they had used, Robert Bromberg.

Mr. Bromberg was an attorney in Cincinnati who had previously headed the section of the IRS that dealt with applications by medical organizations to become tax-exempt, and he now seemed to have a franchise in the business. He would work with a group to see that it met all the IRS requirements. Then, when it met his standards, the client was almost assured of approval. Mr. Bromberg had a different method of dealing with the accounts receivable issue. He would have the group come into compliance and operate as a nonprofit for a few years and then apply for 501(c)(4) status retroactively and 501(c)(3) going forward.[215] Mr. Holets and I met with Mr. Bromberg in the St. Paul Embassy Suites on November 10, 1988, to discuss the process and his evaluation of the Olmsted Medical Group's situation. We reported to the board on November 22 and asked our corporate attorney James Platt to draft the needed resolutions and changes to the articles of incorporation. The Clinic was strongly supportive of our becoming nonprofit, and Mr. Holets and I spent the afternoon of December 21 with Greg Orwall, the head of Mayo Clinic's legal department, getting advice and freely plagiarizing their bylaws. We discussed the process further with the board

---

[215] The main difference is that 501(c)(3) corporations can accept tax-deductible contributions and use tax-exempt financing. Both are exempt from federal corporate income tax.

and shareholders, and at a special meeting on December 27, 1988, the shareholders unanimously adopted the amendments.

Dr. Wente's vision of nonprofit status was coming true. The Olmsted Medical Group was now officially organized for charitable, educational, and scientific purposes, a major step in its metamorphosis. Dr. Wente says that he had thought of the Olmsted Medical Group's becoming nonprofit as far back as 1956, but that it was not possible at that time. In 1974, he proposed selling the Olmsted Medical Group to a new nonprofit entity related to, but not part of, the Mayo Clinic. As the Olmsted Medical Group had recognized in its recent mission and vision statements, its incorporation and various restructurings showed that the organization was gaining a life and importance of its own as an institution, greater than just a group of doctors who might come and go. Nonprofit status could help to solidify that permanence, which would be beneficial for patients and employees.

**

The increasing use of computerized tomography (CT) scans and the number of patients who had to be referred outside the Olmsted Medical Group and hospital suggested that the hospital could afford its own CT scanner. However, a detailed financial analysis showed that a CT scanner could not be justified at that time, and the Olmsted Medical Group considered the possibility of a joint venture with the Albert Lea Medical Group for a mobile CT unit. While the joint CT venture with the Albert Lea Medical Group did not prove to be feasible, the Olmsted Medical Group did reach an agreement with Albert Lea in December to jointly purchase a mobile mammography unit to serve our seven branch clinics and their six. The new unit increased the number of women in those communities who received the recommended screening and demonstrated the feasibility of joint ventures with other clinics.

With the new emergency department now open, the hospital asked that it be staffed around the clock, seven days a week. On weekdays, only about three patients a day were visiting the emergency department, so it was not financially feasible for the Olmsted Medical Group to assign a dedicated doctor there during those times. There was an Olmsted Medical Group internist in the hospital on medical service and an obstetrician, and other doctors could be called over from the Olmsted Medical Group as needed.

This arrangement did not satisfy the hospital or the involved doctors, and 24-hour staffing was started in July after the hospital helped cover part of the Olmsted Medical Group's losses for a time.

To improve access for patients, the pediatrics department started to hold clinics on Saturday mornings in February 1987, and they were quite busy. To improve services further, a special desk was established to expedite insurance and employment exams, and plans were made for an occupational medicine department headed by Dr. Larry Grubbs, who was interested in getting additional training in the area.

Branch clinic expansion continued with requests from the communities of Byron and Elgin in early 1987. Byron was the more promising location and planning was begun for a clinic, which opened in September 1988. The Spring Valley practice of Drs. Roland Matson[216] and Brad Westra joined the Olmsted Medical Group on November 1, 1987, expanding its service area further south. Chatfield Mayor Charles Pavlish approached the Olmsted Medical Group in December about opening a clinic there so that the community would have a full-time doctor, which we agreed to do. The Chatfield branch clinic took shape when the Olmsted Medical Group leased and remodeled a three-story building that had been a hotel, then a bank. The clinic opened on November 17, 1988. The old bank vault made the state's most secure drug cabinet.

The second year of the growth plan continued in 1987 with another orthopedist, Dr. Glenn Johnson, who joined Dr. Peter Frechette in February. He had trained at Mayo Clinic and then served in the Air Force in Alaska. He fell in love with Alaska, purchased a Piper Cub with floats and skis, and planned to join an orthopedics group in Anchorage. In 1986, the Alaskan economy collapsed, and his group was laying off rather than hiring. The Olmsted Medical Group had tried to recruit Dr. Johnson before he joined the Air Force and was happy to get a second chance. Dr. Johnson was an amateur radio operator, and enlisted Dr. Tom Peyla, a fellow ham, to help him erect a roof antenna on the main clinic building so he could have a radio in his office. This was without the knowledge or permission of the administration. One day Mr. Holets happened to look up through the third floor skylight and saw the antenna sticking up. It stayed up throughout Dr. Johnson's tenure.[217]

---

[216] Dr. Matson died Jan. 21, 2008, three days after this was written.
[217] Peyla, T.L. Interview, Sep. 18, 2008.

Dr. Wente retired at the end of 1987 and was honored at a party on January 8, 1988, at the Kahler Hotel. I told him I would say only a couple of words. The words were "vision" and "energy," which formed the basis for my speech. Dr. Wente was a true visionary, innovator, and medical entrepreneur, ahead of his time in many ways; and he had the energy, enthusiasm, and persistence to make his visions happen. He created a medical group that was one of the first to be incorporated and to provide benefits for all employees, and to have computerized business systems, a patient education department, a medical director, professional administration, rural branch clinics, and formal accreditation. He also promoted the attitudes and culture that have continued to lead the organization. Dr. Wente is a strong supporter of Lourdes High School, so as a retirement gift, the board of directors established the Harold A. Wente scholarship for a graduating Lourdes senior planning a career in medicine.

In March 1988, the Olmsted Medical Group board decided to conduct a new community needs assessment to follow up on the 1980 Berkowitz study. The new study confirmed that the Olmsted Medical Group's most attractive feature was free street-level parking, a finding that has now dropped off the list of the top five reasons that patients visit the Olmsted Medical Center, being replaced by convenience and access. To improve communications with patients and to keep them informed of Olmsted Medical Group changes, publication of a quarterly patient newsletter, *HealthNotes*, began in March.

As 1988 ended, the deliberate growth plan was well on its way to being accomplished. The Olmsted Medical Group had 48 physicians, a podiatrist, and three psychologists; and it had completed successful building projects and opened seven branch clinics to serve the surrounding communities. The Olmsted Medical Group now began to concentrate on other issues including integration and consolidation of existing facilities and services, and improved efficiency and quality.

Three more physicians had been hired to start the next year, including Dr. Noel Peterson, the Olmsted Medical Group's first urologist. Dr. Peterson is a native Iowan who graduated from Drake University and started graduate school at the University of Minnesota in biochemistry. This being the Vietnam era, he enlisted in the Navy in 1969 as he was about to be drafted. After he had spent three years in microbiology research at the Bethesda Naval Hospital, the Navy thought he could become a good physician, so it sent him to the University of Iowa for medical school, followed by a residency at the San Diego Naval Medical Center. By 1989, he had served twenty years in the Navy and was interested in joining a private practice. The Olmsted Medical Group was looking for future leaders, and Dr. Peterson proved to be a good fit for the organization.

Glenn Johnson, our Alaska refugee orthopedist, found a position in Bemidji, which was as close to Alaska as he could find, complete with a house on a lake where he could dock his plane. He left in April, but helped us recruit a friend from residency. Bob Kurland, the son of Len Kurland, the Mayo Clinic epidemiologist, had been practicing orthopedics in Milwaukee and joined us May 1. He has been the linchpin of the department ever since.

The Olmsted Medical Group received more requests for new branch clinics in several communities, but declined offers from Lake City, Waseca, and Kenyon. In August 1989, a community group from Preston approached the Olmsted Medical Group with a proposal to open a clinic there. Dr. John Nehring in Preston was moving to Harmony, and although Dr. Sauer was still in Preston, there was a need that the Olmsted Medical Group could fill. Increases in patient visits in Hayfield and Pine Island necessitated increases in size for those two branch clinics, which was accomplished by building new offices for both practices since expansion at their existing sites was not feasible.

At about this time, a community in Portugal contacted the Olmsted Medical Group about opening a clinic in that country. The board thought that Southwestern Europe might be a nice place for retreats but, as it was a bit far for patients to come to the Olmsted Community Hospital, a firm decision was made to leave the international arena to our neighbor.

At the end of 1989, the Mayo Clinic announced the closure of the Methodist Hospital emergency department and the opening of an after-hours clinic at the Baldwin building. The Olmsted Medical Group was concerned that the Olmsted Community Hospital's already crowded emergency department might be inundated, or that Mayo Clinic's evening clinic would take away patients. With the extended hours for pediatrics already proving to be successful, the board decided to expand the service to include family medicine as well, to provide a convenient and less expensive option for Olmsted Medical Group patients and to reduce the potential for overcrowding at the emergency department. CT usage continued to increase, and it now appeared reasonable for the hospital or the Olmsted Medical Group to purchase a scanner within a year. Mr. Holets and I discussed a possible location for the scanner with the radiologists, Dr. Kurowski, and Mr. Cartney, so that the desired space would not be used for something else in the meantime.

The Olmsted Medical Group's attorney, Mr. Bromberg, continued to work on attaining tax-exempt status and sent periodic suggestions or instructions. A public advisory committee was needed to ensure that the Olmsted Medical Group provided the needed public service, that there was no private inurement, and that physicians were not overpaid. Mr. Holets had talked for some time about gathering a group of local business leaders to advise the Olmsted Medical Group and to act as a sounding board for ideas, and this group could serve as the public advisory committee for applying for nonprofit status. The bylaws were changed in August; the committee was appointed in October and met for the first time in November. The members were Lance Davenport, president of Norwest Bank SE Minnesota; Tom Bergsland, president of Electroassembly Inc.; Charlie Pavlish, mayor of Chatfield; Jim Rian, a retired accountant with McGladrey & Pullen; and Bill Tointon, president of McGhee & Betts and also president of the Olmsted Community Hospital board of directors. The committee proved to be very helpful in its role and was a significant contributor to the nonprofit application process.

In January 1990, Mr. Bromberg suggested that the Olmsted Medical Group start a charitable foundation to make its charitable purpose more explicit. By July, the Olmsted Medical and Health Care Foundation was established. The board of directors consisted of the existing public advisory committee members, plus Drs. Garber and Stenberg, Mr. Holets, and me. The first meeting was in October, and in December 1990, the foundation received 501(c)(3) status. The Olmsted Medical Group contributed to the foundation and encouraged individual physicians to do so as well.

The new Hayfield branch clinic building was completed in early April 1990, and construction began immediately afterward on the Pine Island clinic, which opened in late summer. Construction crews broke ground in September for an addition and remodeling of the Spring Valley building. The Olmsted Medical Group continued to believe that a Northwest Rochester branch clinic would be needed within a few years and started a search for a good location. Planning to finish the remaining shelled-in portion of the third floor of the main clinic for internal medicine was begun, with construction to start at the beginning of 1991.

The Olmsted Medical Group's internal medicine department had enjoyed an excellent relationship with Mayo Clinic's cardiologists for some years, and the cardiologists had been doing echocardiograms in the internal medicine department. In September 1991, the cardiologists began doing consultations at the Olmsted Medical Group as well. The presence of the visiting cardiologists helped to cement the Olmsted Medical Group's cordial and collaborative relationships with the Mayo Clinic. The Olmsted Medical Group also contracted with the Minneapolis Clinic of Neurology to provide neurology services to establish a practice that would be ready for Dr. James Smith, a Mayo Clinic neurology fellow, who would join the Olmsted Medical Group in July 1991 after his training was completed.

By the summer of 1990, surgeons in the U.S. were beginning to perform laparoscopic cholecystectomies, removing the gall bladder through a scope instead of through a large incision in the abdominal wall. Dr. Branch and I received training in this technique and did the first cases at the Olmsted Community Hospital that fall. Dr. Branch soon began doing other laparoscopic procedures as well. Our experience with videoendoscopy and colonoscopy made our transition to laparoscopic surgery much easier than that of most surgeons. Today, a substantial portion of surgery is done laparoscopically.

The Olmsted Medical Group began considering another revolutionary technology in 1990. I was asked to join a group of four or five doctors to work with the Olmsted Medical Group's computer service firm CyCare as it developed an electronic medical record. CyCare was later sold to another company, and some of the principals started InteGreat Systems, which developed the electronic medical record system that the Olmsted Medical Center clinics now use. Olmsted Medical Group representatives visited clinics with electronic medical records, further stimulating our interest in computerizing records. However, an electronic medical record was not implemented until 2002 due to the technical difficulties and expense involved.

The Olmsted Medical Group began to prepare for an electronic medical record, though, by installing a digital dictation system, with transcribed and printed notes instead of handwritten notes in patient charts. The transcribed files were then saved in electronic format for eventual loading into a future computerized record. When the electronic record was finally implemented, it was populated with several years of notes, making it much more useful right from the beginning.

Negotiations with Dr. Kurowski about a CT scanner and its location continued. An ideal unfinished area across from the hospital X-ray department had been located, and by June, Mr. Etbauer had data that showed CT utilization had increased to the point of financial viability. The presence of a CT scanner at the hospital would be a great convenience for both hospital and clinic patients because they would not have to be transferred or referred to St. Marys or the Mayo Clinic for the test. The Olmsted Medical Group presented the CT information to Dr. Kurowski and asked him to discuss it with the hospital board.

The Olmsted Medical Group's successful recruiting program brought in increasing numbers of family physicians. Family medicine was a still a new specialty in the process of defining itself, and there were some differences of opinion within the department regarding the differing needs and issues of the main clinic physicians in Rochester and the branch clinic physicians. To improve the management and operation of the family medicine department and to ensure that the needs of patients and physicians at all clinics were met, it was decided to divide family medicine into three sections: Rochester and north and south branch clinics. The emergency department was also separated from family medicine since the long-term plan was to move to full-time emergency physicians. As the clinical departments grew in size along with the growth of the Olmsted Medical Group, they tended to develop their own interests, which were sometimes inconsistent with those of the organization. In order to align the interests of all of the departments, the department chair positions were strengthened, and the Olmsted Medical Group provided administrative training and assigned an administrator to each department, thus improving communication and coordination.

As the Olmsted Medical Group grew, it became more attractive to physicians. Nevertheless, recruiting continued to be a major effort as the Olmsted Medical Group tried to keep up with the demand for services. Psychiatrist Dr. Bob Nesheim, who had gotten into sled dog racing, moved to Duluth at the end of 1989, but helped recruit Dr. Larry Peterson away from Gundersen to replace him in January. Dr. Peterson is also an excellent cartoonist and caricaturist, and for several years he designed t-shirts for our summer picnics. Dr. Craig

Chambers, a Mayo Clinic-trained internist originally from Rochester, came to the Olmsted Medical Group from Marshfield, Wisconsin, in May, and was a great addition for those who don't mind a steady stream of puns.

An important addition in July 1990 was Dr. Roy Yawn. Dr. Yawn is a native Georgian, who graduated from the Massachusetts Institute of Technology, where his wife Barbara was also a student. Both graduated from the University of Missouri Medical School. Dr. Roy Yawn completed an internal medicine residency at the University of Minnesota while Barbara studied family medicine there. They practiced for 14 years in Worthington, Minnesota, where he became president of the local clinic. Barbara became interested in research and came to Rochester to work on research projects at Mayo Clinic while she studied for a master's degree in clinical research design and statistics from the University of Michigan, and Roy joined the Olmsted Medical Group's internal medicine department. Dr. Roy Yawn went on to serve as department chair for 10 years, as a member of the board of governors, and then as president and CEO of the Olmsted Medical Center.

Since its beginning, the Olmsted Medical Group had had the highest percentage of women physicians of any multispecialty group in the country. This was partly because of the presence of a number of Mayo Clinic spouses. Also, the Olmsted Medical Group was one of very few that allowed part-time practice, and it may have been the only one that allowed part-time physicians to be shareholders. For several years, women physicians, including one who worked part time, held a majority of the Olmsted Medical Group's board seats. Nonetheless, there was some concern about the loss of several women physicians in a short period of time, and a gender-issues task force was appointed to study the issues faced by women physicians at the Olmsted Medical Group, such as conflicts between work and family needs, cultural and societal pressures, pay, benefits, work hours, and call duties. The task force found that many of the issues were more generational than gender-related, and the Olmsted Medical Group made changes to involve more of the younger doctors. To make the Olmsted Medical Group more attractive to women physicians, training programs about sensitivity to women's issues and a new sexual harassment policy were developed.

At the invitation of Lance Davenport, I spoke at the Rochester Downtown Rotary Club on January 10, 1991. I talked mostly about the history of the Olmsted Medical Group, its growth, and quality improvement initiatives. I also mentioned the need for a CT scanner. I noted that we had sent more than 600 patients to Mayo Clinic for this procedure the previous year and that the number of referrals was increasing steadily. In addition, I discussed the Olmsted Medical Group's intent to become nonprofit and the case for a merger between the Olmsted Medical Group and the Olmsted Community Hospital. The two organizations were a de facto system, but with two boards and administrations and different philosophies. The Olmsted Medical Group was growth oriented, while the county operated with fixed revenues and was oriented toward controlling expenses. Following this meeting, I was asked to speak about these issues at a Kiwanis Club, a group in Chatfield, and several other civic groups.

* * *

The Olmsted County Board made organizational changes in late 1990 that led to the merger of the Olmsted Community Hospital and the county health department, forming the Olmsted Community Health Center. The new combined board of directors asked me to address its first meeting on January 30, 1991. I talked about the Olmsted Medical Group's history, present activities, and conversion to nonprofit status. I addressed the need for a CT scanner, a proposal that still had not been presented to the hospital board. I also shared the Olmsted Medical Group's view that the community would be better served by a merger of the hospital and the Olmsted Medical Group. The delay in resolving the CT issue was a prime example of the need for a merger of the Olmsted Community Hospital and the Olmsted Medical Group.

The Olmsted Medical Group updated the CT usage and financial data for Dr. Kurowski to present at the February 1991 board meeting, but the item did not appear on the agenda until the April 24 meeting. Dr. Karen Lundquist, a Olmsted Medical Group radiologist, and a radiology technician attended the meeting to represent our point of view, but the subject was not raised. Mr. Cartney presented the proposal at the June board meeting, but he was simply instructed to gather more information for a future meeting. I was asked to speak at that same June meeting about the relationship of the Olmsted Medical Group to the hospital and its medical staff, which the Olmsted Medical Group nearly entirely comprised. I again advocated for a merger of the Olmsted Medical Group and the hospital, along the lines of Mayo Clinic's relationship with its hospitals, when the Olmsted Medical Group attained tax-exempt status.

The Olmsted Medical Group continued to urge action on the CT scanner in subsequent meetings with Dr. Kurowski and Mr. Cartney. There were other issues, too, such as increased space for the obstetrics clinic and additional emergency department staffing that required cooperation between the two institutions. Dr. Kurowski understood the need for the two organizations to be better coordinated, and the Olmsted Medical Group succeeded in getting the hospital and Olmsted Medical Group clinical departments aligned so that, for the most part, the same physician department chairs were appointed at both places. Dr. Kurowski suggested that the Olmsted Medical Group president serve as the hospital staff president, but I thought it more appropriate for the president to be an ex officio member of the executive committee. The Olmsted Medical Group continued to urge the purchase of a CT scanner to assist in recruiting radiologists and to increase the hospital's revenue.

* * *

The Olmsted Medical Group's application for tax exemption was transferred in March 1991 from the Chicago regional office to the Washington IRS headquarters. Mr. Holets met with Mr. Bromberg in Cincinnati in December to review additional information requested by the IRS. In early February 1992, Mr. Bromberg informed the Olmsted Medical Group that its application had passed the first reviewer, but that before it got to the final review, the Office of the General Counsel of the IRS had decided to do a study of the whole issue of tax exemption for medical groups. That would delay the ruling at least until the summer of 1992.

In August 1991, Dr. Barbara Yawn asked the Olmsted Medical Group to participate in two studies she was conducting at Mayo Clinic in conjunction with her master's degree program in research. Two months later, she asked about doing research for the Olmsted Medical Group on a contract basis after she completed her master's degree. The next January, she became an independent contractor for the Olmsted Medical Group's charitable foundation, and became an employee of the Olmsted Medical Group the following year. The establishment of a research department at the Olmsted Medical Group assisted with its effort to attain nonprofit status, and cemented relationships with the Rochester Epidemiology Project housed at Mayo Clinic. The Olmsted Medical Group research department was unique among medical groups of this size and even more unusual because it was largely self-supporting through grants.

At the regular meeting between the Olmsted Medical Group and Mayo Clinic leaders in September, the Mayo Clinic representatives seemed cool to the idea of the hospital or the Olmsted Medical Group obtaining a CT scanner, and said that the Olmsted Medical Group's new extended hours and acute illness department made it seem more competitive and less complementary to Mayo Clinic. I pointed out that, as the Mayo Clinic and other academic medical centers pushed the cutting edge of medical practice into new territory, tests and procedures that had once been cutting edge became standard practice for other clinics and hospitals. This is good for patients as well as medical practices. The Olmsted Medical Group would be broadening its scope as Mayo Clinic broadened its, and they saw my point. Relationships between the two organizations were further strengthened when the Olmsted Medical Group agreed to become a primary teaching site for Mayo Clinic's ultrasonographer training program.

As the number of physicians at the Olmsted Medical Group had more than doubled, along with more specialties and branch locations, Dr. Gary Oftedahl was becoming overwhelmed as medical director. The board decided at the end of 1991 to divide the medical directorship into two positions. Dr. James Garber would become coordinator of physician resources, and Dr. Oftedahl was appointed coordinator of quality management. Dr. Barbara Yawn became coordinator of clinical research. Dr. David Lundberg, who had been on the staff of the Franciscan Skemp family practice residency in La Crosse, Wisconsin, was recruited to start an acute illness department in January 1992.

* * *

In January 1992, Dr. Kurowski presented a proposal that the Olmsted Medical Group cover all the indirect expenses for the CT scanner and up to $50,000 in losses. The Olmsted Medical Group did not agree with the first provision since indirect revenues were not included in the proposal, but covering losses was not a problem since by now we believed there would be none. Dr. Kurowski presented his projections to the Olmsted Community Health Center board on January 29, showing $73,000 in losses in the first two years, followed by a profit. The board authorized him to develop specifications for a scanner. On June 24, after the Olmsted Medical Group made a formal presentation and agreed to cover losses, the Community Health Center board authorized the lease-purchase of a General Electric CT scanner. The county board confirmed this on July 7, a little over two years after the Olmsted Medical Group had determined that a CT scanner was financially feasible. Contracts were awarded in late October for remodeling the previously reserved unfinished space in the hospital for the scanner, which finally became operational in January 1993.

In 1993, Dr. Barbara Yawn established the organization's Institutional Review Board to review research proposals for safety and regulatory compliance, which is especially important for receiving government research grants. Colleen Gau, our patient educator, left nursing to earn a PhD in the history of clothing, so Dr. Barbara Yawn also became director of education as well as research. The Olmsted Medical Group recognized the need to prepare its future leaders, and encouraged Dr. Noel Peterson to enter a program at the University of Wisconsin to earn a master's degree in medical management. Dr. Peterson completed the program and was appointed medical director to succeed Dr. James Garber. Dr. Peterson was also elected to the Minnesota Medical Association board of trustees, replacing Dr. Tom Peyla. Dr. Peyla had become the Olmsted Medical Group's first physician to become a Minnesota Medical Association delegate to the American Medical Association, where he served 10 years.

In March 1993, the Olmsted Medical Group learned that Dr. Brid MacBride, a family practitioner who had recently been hired, could not be licensed because the Minnesota Board of Medical Practice did not recognize her British medical training. The Board of Medical Practice required at least two years in a U.S. residency program before it would issue a license. Undeterred and following Dr. Wente's example of ingenuity in solving difficult problems, the Olmsted Medical Group decided to establish a residency program. By November, the Board of Medical Practice approved the plan, and Dr. MacBride was enrolled. She completed the program with excellent reviews on October 30, 1995, and joined the staff one month later. She was the best resident we have ever had.

In late November 1992, Mr. Bromberg informed the Olmsted Medical Group that the IRS was concerned about its retaining the professional association structure, even with the public advisory committee. The IRS was concerned that the changes the Olmsted Medical Group had made could be reversed too easily. Mr. Bromberg thought the Olmsted Medical Group would need to reincorporate as a not-for-profit corporation. An action of the Olmsted Medical Group shareholders was necessary to proceed, and a special shareholders meeting was held on December 10, 1992. The shareholders unanimously approved proceeding along that path if necessary. Mr. Bromberg, our primary corporate attorney James Platt, Mr. Holets, and I met with IRS officials in Washington on December 17. The IRS officials were very pleasant and supportive, and they seemed impressed that, aside from returning the shareholders' original investment, the Olmsted Medical Group's shareholders were giving, rather than selling, the assets to the new nonprofit entity and would not receive a charitable tax deduction. We agreed to create a new board of trustees with eight public members and five physicians elected by the medical staff as internal trustees. The five physicians would also constitute the board of governors. The trustees would have the public oversight function, similar to the current public advisory committee. The governors would act essentially as the present Olmsted Medical Group directors, setting physician and operational policies. On returning from Washington, Mr. Platt quickly filed new articles of incorporation with the state of Minnesota before the end of the year. A board of trustees was established, including Messrs. Bergsland, Davenport, and Pavlish from the public advisory committee; Bill Pudwell, president of the Olmsted Community Health Center board; Karen Nagle, president of Rochester Community and Technical College; Barbara McLane, an IBM executive; Dan Berndt, an attorney with Dunlap & Seeger; and Dr. Tom Sitzer, a pediodontist and long-time member of the Olmsted Community Hospital staff. Lance Davenport became the chairman of the board of trustees. The board reviewed the draft bylaws in February 1993 and decided to add the chief administrative officer and the medical director[218] to the board of governors.

On April 30, 1993, the new application for tax exemption was filed with the IRS. In August, the Olmsted Medical Group received two letters from the IRS, both dated August 6, 1993. The first stated that the Olmsted Medical Group, P.A. had been determined to be a 501(c)(4) organization as of January 1, 1988, and was eligible for refund of taxes since that time. The second letter stated that the Olmsted Medical Group, Inc. was determined to be a 501(c)(3) organization, effective December 30, 1992. The shareholders held a special meeting on August 30, at which Mr. Platt, Tom Holets, and I again explained, in great detail, the legal and financial ramifications of the conversion. A resolution was then passed unanimously to transfer the assets

---

[218] The coordinator of physician resources was again the medical director.

and liabilities from the professional association to the new corporation and to dissolve the professional association as of October 1, 1993.

The board of trustees met the following evening and accepted the transfer. The notice of intent to dissolve the professional association was signed on September 30 and filed with the Secretary of State on October 4. A news conference and ceremonial signing of the documents was held the next day. At the news conference, I pointed out that, "As the Olmsted Medical Group has grown and become more complex, it has become an important community resource, far outweighing the importance of any of its physicians. With the Olmsted Community Hospital, with which it is completely interdependent, it constitutes a healthcare system with revenues of $38 million, 550 employees and a $17.5 million payroll." I further stated: "It has become apparent that a physician-owned corporation is no longer the most appropriate or effective structure for the group. Accordingly, the doctor-owners of the Olmsted Medical Group have voted unanimously to give the Olmsted Medical Group to a new not-for-profit corporation. No one actually owns the Olmsted Medical Group now, but the board of trustees holds it in trust for the benefit of the public." The *Post-Bulletin* carried a news article that evening and on October 12 printed a large, very complimentary article, headlined: "An act of charity, community spirit." It followed two days later with a laudatory editorial.

The restructuring of the Olmsted Medical Group was undoubtedly made easier by the local example of the Mayo Clinic, where we all had friends and some had spouses or had trained. The culture established by Dr. Wente and his early colleagues was at least as big a factor. And the ongoing history of the Olmsted Medical Group seemed to lead inexorably in that direction.

Chapter 10
The Olmsted Medical Center

The possibility of a merger with the Olmsted Community Hospital was the last of our reasons for taking the Olmsted Medical Group nonprofit. In 1988, that had seemed like a long shot. We had three primary motives. First, the organization would be able to retain earnings without having them doubly taxed, which would allow the organization to grow and increase its IRS services. Also, the Olmsted Medical Group would be able to own real estate without needing a separate partnership. And it would have access to tax-exempt financing. We immediately began to pursue both of these last two goals.

Mr. Holets started working up a presentation for the IRS to get an exemption to allow the purchase of the Ninth Street building from Olmsted Medical Properties.[219] The application was filed on December 15, 1993, and was approved in just six weeks. The building was appraised at $5.3 million and the agreed purchase price was $4.391 million, which made it easy for the IRS to approve.

The Olmsted Medical Group hired bond counsel and met with Cain Brothers, a New York underwriter, that would issue and market our tax-exempt securities, which would be City of Rochester recapitalization bonds. Mr. Holets discussed the bond issue with the city administrator and on March 21, 1994, the city council held a public hearing, and then unanimously approved it. The Putnam Group bought the entire $6 million issue. The success of the bond issue was a credit to the Olmsted Medical Group's improved financial management and position. It was clear that the organization had the financial discipline to make good use of the funds and to repay the debt.

In April 1994, Dr. Werner Kaese retired after almost 35 years as the heart and soul of the department of obstetrics and gynecology. He said that it seemed like no time at all to him. As we were talking at his retirement party, he said to me, "How can I be retiring? I just finished medical school."

The Olmsted Medical Group continued to grow, including a new generation of relatives of Elaine Wente. Dr. Martha Bowman, a distant cousin through

---

[219] As these were related parties, such a transaction was prohibited without prior IRS approval.

her mother's side, joined the internal medicine department in 1994, and Dr. John Cierzan followed in 1996. Dr. Cierzan is another relative of Elaine, a first cousin of Dr. Bowman, and a Lourdes classmate of Teresa Wente, Hal and Elaine's youngest daughter.

There continued to be activity in the branch clinics. The Chatfield clinic became overloaded and could not take more patients, leading to a renewed interest in opening a clinic in Preston. A market study in the summer of 1994 was favorable and Dr. Stephanie Jakim agreed to staff an office there. The local bank had an available building site, and the Preston clinic opened in October 1995. Dr. Al Risser, the last of the original hospital staff, retired at the end of June 1994 after 56 years of practice in Stewartville. He transferred his medical records to the Olmsted Medical Group, and the Stewartville branch clinic expanded into the space we had loaned him.

In the spring of 1995, I was asked to join the board of the Midwest Medical Insurance Company (MMIC). This was my most interesting and enjoyable outside activity because of my interest in insurance and risk management. MMIC had grown to insure physicians in four states and would soon become the leading insurer in a six-state area. It had developed a strong risk-management program to help physicians avoid problems that could lead to malpractice claims.

A new tradition for the Olmsted Medical Group began on July 12, 1995, with the first Founders Day dinner. This event arose from an idea that occurred to Dr. Garber when he attended a similar event for another organization. The purpose of the annual dinner was to show appreciation to Dr. Wente and all of the people who had contributed to the growth and development of the Olmsted Medical Group. The idea was also consistent with the concept of creating and passing along an organizational history and mythology. The dinner was to be held on the Wednesday evening closest to July 15, the day on which Dr. Wente opened his first office, and the location was Michael's Restaurant, the scene of many meetings of the Olmsted Medical Group's doctors. Retired and senior practicing physicians were invited so that they could maintain their connections and friendships. The dinner allowed retirees to be kept informed of current events at the Olmsted Medical Group, while also serving as an opportunity to promote contributions and bequests. The dinner was a great success, and the annual event continues to the present time, although at a new location that can accommodate a larger gathering.

By the time the Olmsted Medical Group achieved its tax-exempt status, the possibility of a merger with the Olmsted Community Hospital had been openly discussed for almost six years. It was also becoming apparent to many people that the hospital-health department merger was not working. The two lacked synergy and, while the mission statements of the hospital and health department used nearly the same words, they were used in different contexts and had different meanings.[220] Mr. Holets met with Mr. Devlin in November 1993 about establishing a joint task force to review the benefits and pitfalls of a closer relationship between the Olmsted Medical Group and the hospital. Mr. Devlin reported that the county was still moving toward a more thorough integration of the hospital and health department. But at the county's suggestion, on January 5, 1994, board members of the Olmsted Community Health Center and the Olmsted Medical Group, as well as representatives of the county government, met in the Olmsted Medical Group's library. The purpose of the meeting was "to discuss the possibility of undertaking an evaluative process for the purpose of identifying potential advantages of a closer working relationship between the Olmsted Community Health Center and Olmsted Medical Group." Six task forces composed of employees from both the Community Health Center and the Olmsted Medical Group were formed to look at various functions, to break them down into components, and to report on which ones might be best served by closer cooperation, joint ventures, consolidation, or complete merger.

The Integration Exploration Steering Committee reviewed the interim task force reports on July 18. Mr. Cartney, the acting administrator of the hospital, reported that the teams were enthusiastic and had identified much duplication and redundancy. All the teams were "certainly behind the idea of consolidating certain services. If pressed, in fact, many of the teams might be in favor of a full-fledged merger of the organizations, or at least of the Olmsted Community Hospital and the Olmsted Medical Group." There was further discussion about whether the health department should be included in a merger. Mr. Holets reported that some of the teams could not answer all their questions without outside assistance and recommended hiring a consultant to review certain financial issues. The organizations agreed to share the costs and to engage Deloitte & Touche, the hospital's auditor.

---

[220] Wellik M., Interview, February 11, 2008.

The final team reports were reviewed on August 17 and unanimously favored a merger of the Olmsted Medical Group and the Olmsted Community Hospital as the most effective solution. The consultants reported on the same day that there were neither financial barriers to a merger nor any from the hospital or Medical Group bond agreements. They were then asked to examine possible organizational structures and reported those findings to the steering committee on January 9, 1995. Since a county department was not permitted to merge with a private corporation, the hospital had to be acquired either by the Olmsted Medical Group corporation or a new one. Recent changes in federal regulations made it preferable to have the Olmsted Medical Group corporation survive, with the county appointing some board members. Hospital and county representatives agreed with this proposal, and the consultants then developed methods for transfer of the hospital's assets.

Special legislation to allow the county to transfer the hospital to a private medical group would be needed. Olmsted Medical Group, hospital, and county representatives met with area legislators in St. Paul on February 9 to explain the plan and to obtain their support. Rep. Greg Davids from Preston summed up what had been said about the de facto system when he asked, "Does anybody think it hasn't already happened?" Sen. Sheila Kiscaden and Rep. Fran Bradley introduced the bill, which county attorney Ray Schmitz had helped to draft. Rep. Tom Huntley of Duluth helped on the Democratic side, because St. Louis County wanted to do something jointly with one of its hospitals and they thought the action would set a useful precedent. The recent privatization of St. Paul Ramsey Hospital[221] was a useful precedent also. There were some concerns about the impact on the hospital employees' retirement plan, but these were allayed, and the bill passed the house unanimously on March 29.[222] The Senate followed suit on April 22[223] and sent the bill to Governor Carlson, who signed it.

The final hurdles to complete the merger were agreement on a contract between the parties and approval by the county commissioners and the Olmsted Medical Group board of trustees. The county board held its first public hearing on the merger proposal on February 28. Three more hearings followed, and nearly all of the attendees had connections to either

[221] Now Regions Medical Center.
[222] *Post-Bulletin*, March 30, 1995.
[223] *Post-Bulletin*, April 22, 1995.

the hospital or the Olmsted Medical Group. The Olmsted Medical Group preferred that the merger occur at the end of the year and a number of operational details had to be settled, so there was some pressure on the county to move forward. Negotiations between the Olmsted Medical Group and Olmsted County began on August 8, and an agreement on the basic issues was reached the next week. The proposed plan was reviewed on September 19 and 26 to be sure that each party understood the details. There was a final meeting at the Minneapolis office of Dorsey & Whitney, the county's attorneys, on October 3 to finalize the contracts.

The merger agreement stipulated that the board of trustees of the corporation, to be renamed the Olmsted Medical Center, would consist of the five members elected by the employed physicians of the Olmsted Medical Group, five public members appointed by the county and five more public members elected by the first 10. The Olmsted Medical Center would lease the hospital facilities until the hospital bonds were paid off in 10 years. At that time, it could purchase the hospital for one dollar, the county would withdraw, and the ten public trustees would become self-perpetuating. The county would receive the $2 million that it calculated as its previous investment in the hospital, and the remaining hospital funds would be transferred to the Olmsted Medical Center as operating capital. There were provisions for charity care, protection for employees, and a requirement to maintain an open medical staff available to any appropriately qualified community physicians.

The county board held its last public hearing on October 10, at which I presented a brief history of the Olmsted Medical Group, the nonprofit conversion, and the boards and their functions. I pointed out that the physician trustees had exactly the same responsibilities as the public trustees, which are to act in the interests of the public, not the physicians. I then briefly made the case for merger. The Olmsted Medical Group board of trustees unanimously approved the merger on October 18. Two days later, the *Post-Bulletin* ran an editorial advocating changes to the agreement. The editor feared that the Olmsted Medical Group would revert to for-profit status in 10 years. My reply was quoted in a news article on October 23 headlined, "OMG Chairman: Hospital will stay nonprofit." I explained that the bond covenants required the Olmsted Medical Group to remain tax-exempt until the bonds were paid in 2019. In reality, it would be virtually impossible for the corporation to revert to private, for-profit status. The county board unanimously approved the merger on October 24, to take effect on January 1, 1996. The closing took place at Dorsey & Whitney's Rochester office on December 12.

The Olmsted Medical Group officially changed its name to Olmsted Medical Center. The clinic trustees were Drs. Branch, Geier, Peyla, Stenberg, and Thauwald. The county appointed as public trustees Commissioners Carol Kamper and Mike Podulke, Mr. Devlin, Tom Ferguson from the Community Health Center board, and Brenda Riggott with the Chamber of Commerce. The other public trustees were Tom Bergsland, Dan Berndt, Lance Davenport, and Karen Nagle from the Olmsted Medical Group board, and Bill Pudwell from both the previous boards and a former county commissioner. Mr. Davenport was elected chairman and Mr. Berndt vice-chairman. Mr. Cartney and Mrs. Brezicka were also added to the board of governors.

There was little time to organize the management team before the first of the year. The decision was made to integrate as much as possible immediately, rather than extending the process over several years. The hospital had relied on the county for a number of support functions and had no human resources department or payroll system. Lois Till-Tarara was assigned to manage human resources, and because the Olmsted Medical Group payroll system was already near capacity, this function was outsourced to ADT. Mr. Holets and Ms. Till-Tarara worked with the county and employee groups to create a merged package of benefits, which was generally better than the previous packages for either group of employees. Terry Nelson from the hospital took charge of accounting. Mr. Cartney took over branch clinic and business office operations, and Karen Brezicka was given charge of clinic as well as hospital nursing and other patient services. Dennis Etbauer headed facilities, equipment, and purchasing. Sue Schuett from the Olmsted Medical Group was in charge of information technology. The radiology departments and laboratories were merged and physical therapy, accounting, and central supply were consolidated at the hospital.

We had planned to retain the names of Olmsted Community Hospital and Olmsted Medical Group and to use Olmsted Medical Center just for the corporate entity. However, on the day the merger became effective, the employees at all facilities showed a great deal of pride by answering the telephone, "Olmsted Medical Center, Hospital," "Olmsted Medical Center, Pine Island" and similar greetings. New hospital and medical staff bylaws would be required before the Joint Commission visit in May. Dr. Roger Lindeman at Virginia Mason, Dr. Frank Riddick at the Ochsner Medical Center in New Orleans, and Dr. Stu Hanson at Park Nicollet were all very helpful in providing information to assist with their preparation. The trustees reviewed the corporate bylaws in March and approved changes to the portions related to the professional staff and auxiliary. The Joint Commission survey in May went very well, and in August, the hospital received full accreditation.

With the merger, the board of governors now received many routine reports, plans, and procedures from the hospital to meet regulatory requirements as well as new business items. In April, a private letter ruling from the IRS stated that the acquisition of the hospital would not adversely affect the Medical Center's tax-exempt status. Surprisingly, the Minnesota Department of Revenue denied a routine application for sales tax exemption for hospital purchases on the grounds that, since the merger, it was no longer a hospital, which was very confusing since they also stated that there was no legal definition of "hospital." Discussions with the Department of Revenue were not helpful, and ultimately legislation was required to avoid our having the state's only hospital subject to sales tax.

Hammel, Green, and Abrahamson, the architects for the hospital's last building program, were engaged to develop a master facilities plan. Hal Henderson, whose company, Construction Collaborative, had designed the Olmsted Medical Group's branch clinics and other remodeling projects, had recently joined Hammel, Green, and Abrahamson and headed a new Rochester office. A similar study of information systems needs and organization was conducted.

A new branch clinic in Wanamingo was acquired after the Zumbrota Clinic closed. The physician's assistant who had been staffing the clinic, Norman Booth, agreed to stay on there as an Olmsted Medical Center employee. The Olmsted Medical Center continued to plan a Northwest Rochester branch clinic. Possible sites were examined, and Mr. Etbauer obtained data about traffic patterns, population density, and other relevant factors in the northwest area. After evaluating 15 potential sites, a location at 43rd Street and the Highway 52 West Frontage Road was purchased for the new clinic.

In September 1996, Joel Rueber, the administrator of Mayo Clinic's family medicine department, gave a talk at the Scott and White Clinic Club, a group of the largest clinics in the country. He described Mayo Clinic's competition with the Olmsted Medical Center. Mayo Clinic's market share in Rochester had been decreasing steadily. They looked at their market demographics and realized patients were bypassing their clinic because they didn't like the parking ramp; Mayo Clinic was also having capacity problems. They were considering creating a clinic in the northwest part of the city to help regain market share there. The title of the talk was "In the Shadow of the Shadow."

Mr. Holets, our administrator for 12 years and a key person in planning and implementing the merger, announced in November that he was leaving in January to join Phycor as administrator of the Lexington Clinic in Kentucky. This was a great disappointment for me since I had greatly enjoyed working with Mr. Holets. We constantly bounced ideas off each other, tore them apart, and reworked the good parts until we couldn't tell anymore whose idea it had originally been. The 12 years that we had worked together were the most productive, rewarding, and enjoyable of my career.

There were more than 60 applicants to replace Mr. Holets, and of these Mark Jenkins, vice president at the Dean Medical Center in Madison, Wisconsin, was selected for the position. He was a graduate of Penn State and a classmate of Mr. Holets in the Iowa master's program. He was bright, personable, and energetic, and came highly recommended. Dr. Branch and I were re-elected to the boards in February 1997. After 13 years as president, I had not planned to run again until Mr. Holets announced his departure. Just one year into the merger, I didn't think that the Olmsted Medical Center should turn over both of those positions for fear of losing momentum and direction.

The trustees were very pleased with the $326,000 in charity care that the Olmsted Medical Center delivered in the first year of the merger, since this was two and a half times the amount the county had asked for. The trustees also became interested in quality improvement reports and comparisons to benchmarks. Dr. Barbara Yawn informed the board that the Olmsted Medical Center's continuing education program for physicians had been accredited and discussed the problems that Minnesota's new privacy law would cause for clinical research.

The Northwest Rochester branch clinic was planned as a 5600-square-foot building and financed with an $800,000 bond issue through the county. Ground breaking was on June 10, 1997. The building was to be partially finished, with an area for later expansion if needed. By the time the clinic opened on December 15, it was already apparent that the expansion would need to be completed by the next July.

Another surprise was in store for the Olmsted Medical Center. On September 15, while I was attending the Minnesota Medical Association annual meeting and visiting with Dr. David Orgel, IBM Rochester's medical director, he casually mentioned IBM's new HMO contract with HealthPartners, for which the Olmsted Medical Center was to be the provider. The Olmsted Medical Center had heard nothing about this; and we learned that IBM Rochester and HealthPartners had only known of it themselves for a few days because the contract had been negotiated at the national level with no local involvement. Open enrollment started October 1, and provisions had not been made for educating the employees about the difference between capitation and indemnity insurance. IBM held a benefits fair on October 2, at which Olmsted Medical Center representatives were able to talk to a small number of employees. The lack of education of how HMOs operate led to much misunderstanding and dissatisfaction among the patients as well as the doctors. While the Olmsted Medical Center was interested in an opportunity to demonstrate its high quality and lower costs through the management of capitated patients, this experiment ultimately failed due to a lack of understanding and support for the concept on the part of employers, patients and doctors. After a few years, the Olmsted Medical Center returned to fee-for-service contracts.

In early 1998, Mr. Jenkins elected to step down as the chief administrative officer, but remained with the organization for an additional year working on special projects. The Olmsted Medical Center resumed its search for a chief administrator and had even more applicants than before, with a wide variety of backgrounds. Dan Marren, an assistant administrator with MeritCare, a large integrated system in Fargo, was selected for the position. He had the most experience in a merged organization and had managed on both the clinic and hospital sides. He had bachelor's and master's degrees from Wichita State and a master of healthcare administration from Notre Dame. Two other important additions to our administrative staff were Troy Stafford, a new chief financial officer, and Sharon Gabrielson, director of nursing.

Like CT, magnetic resonance imaging (MRI) scanning had now become a routine part of medical practice rather than a technique reserved for specialists, and the Olmsted Medical Center thoroughly researched the feasibility of providing this service to its patients. MRI referrals to outside providers were tracked, site visits were made to learn more about the equipment and patient processing, and the financial aspects were examined. A formal proposal to purchase an MRI scanner was presented to the board executive committee on a Tuesday morning. The board of governors endorsed the recommendation that evening and referred it to the board of trustees the next afternoon. The purchase was authorized, and the scanner was ordered on Thursday morning. A process which took more than two years for the CT scanner now took two days, a remarkable improvement due to the merger and consolidation of administrative and governance functions.

The Olmsted Medical Center continued its search for space for its growing volume of patients and staff. The addition of a fourth floor to the main clinic building would meet only the immediate needs, so to acquire the additional space that would be needed, the board elected to exercise the option of taking over the health department's space at the hospital with the required two-year notice to the county. The county agreed and started to plan the current health department building on the campus across the road from the hospital. The Olmsted Medical Center would use the health department space primarily for the obstetrics department, relieving congestion at the main clinic, and allowing more space there for internal medicine, dermatology, and surgery. Construction of the main clinic fourth floor was scheduled to begin in February.

In the late 1990s, the job market was extremely tight, particularly for nurses, and the Olmsted Medical Center raised salaries several times to remain competitive. The hospital nurses were stressed because of staffing shortages despite employing agency nurses from the Twin Cities to supplement the staff. Sue Klenner was asked to form a nursing work group in December 1998 as a quality improvement team, with representatives from each of the nursing units. The work group was given direct access to both the board of governors and the board of trustees and reported to them regularly, helping to improve communications and morale. The work group continued to function until July 2006, when the present nursing council replaced it.

In addition to continued shortages of nurses, other clinical personnel were difficult to recruit because of Mayo Clinic's expansion and need for new staff. For example, Mayo Clinic not only recruited the entire Rochester class of surgical technicians, but all of the class from Grand Forks as well. The Olmsted Medical Center addressed its staffing needs by recruiting interested LPNs and receptionists from our staff and arranging with Rochester Community and Technical College to conduct a special surgical technician training program for them. Sandy Schlachter, an LPN who graduated from the program, still works in the Olmsted Medical Center surgery department.

After the departure of Mr. Marren as chief administrator in November 1999, the Olmsted Medical Center chose Kevin Pitzer, a graduate of the University of Iowa master's program, to fill the position of chief administrative officer. He had worked in Mayo Clinic's administrative trainee program, and then moved to Scottsdale to head patient accounts. He was later in charge of developing Mayo Clinic's primary care network in Scottsdale and was involved in developing the Mayo-John Deere clinics in Moline, Illinois. He returned to Arizona as administrator of the clinics for Scottsdale Healthcare before joining the Olmsted Medical Center.

In April 1999, the board decided to close the Elgin branch clinic, which could not be enlarged, and to move that practice to Plainview. Plainview was a considerably larger town, centrally located in Wabasha County, and a majority of the patients seen at the Elgin clinic actually lived in or closer to Plainview. Construction in Plainview began in May, and the clinic opened in late October with Dr. Dan Pesch and Dr. Tom Peyla, who had moved to a home near Wabasha a few years earlier. Alane Booth, who had recently completed physician's assistant training, joined them. The Elgin building was donated to the community to house its ambulance service.

The Joint Commission surveyed the entire organization in May, spending two days at the hospital, one at the main clinic, and one visiting five branch clinics. The outcome of the survey was very positive, and certification was continued. The Olmsted Medical Center's laboratories were surveyed and certified by the College of American Pathologists.

As the board of governors prepared for upcoming changes in leadership, Dr. Larry Peterson was chosen as medical director for physician personnel and Dr. Gary Oftedahl as medical director for quality improvement. My last annual meeting as president was on February 21, 2000. Drs. Randy Hemann and Noel Peterson were elected clinic trustees, replacing Dr. Branch and me. Dr. Peterson succeeded me as president at the next board of trustees meeting. I was presented with a nice rocking chair with the Olmsted Medical Center logo and my name on the back, and Drs. Stead and Stenberg gave me a bent-shaft canoe paddle to dip in the Boundary Waters. After 20 years on the board and 16 as president, I could get back to being a full-time surgeon. In my last annual report, I quoted from my first one 15 years earlier: "In joining this group practice, we have chosen to be an integrated unit rather than a bunch of individuals sharing an office building. In the face of strong and shifting external stresses we must achieve even greater cohesion and work together in the same direction toward our common goals. We have all heard the famous Chinese curse, 'May you live in interesting times.' There is no doubt that we live in interesting times; whether it is a curse or an exciting adventure is up to us."

For me, it had been the adventure of a lifetime. For the Olmsted Medical Center, many opportunities and challenges remained as the organization moved into the new millennium.

Chapter 11
Into the New Millennium

As the new millennium dawned, Dr. Noel R. Peterson assumed the presidency of the Olmsted Medical Center, well prepared to lead the organization. He was its first physician leader with formal management education, a master's degree in medical management from the University of Wisconsin. Like Dr. John Brodhun, the Olmsted Medical Group's president from 1978 to 1984, Dr. Peterson practiced an inclusive, collegial management style. Dr. Peterson maintained the direction and culture of the organization during a period of continued rapid growth, multiple construction projects, and the implementation of many new services. There were also advances to maintain and improve the quality and convenience of patient care. Dr. Peterson strongly advocated for improved patient safety and provided leadership in that area. Dr. Peterson and the Olmsted Medical Center's boards and management effectively tackled the perennial problems of providing adequate office space to meet patient and staff needs, adding new medical services and technology, quality of care, and patient safety improvements.

The fourth-floor addition at the main clinic was completed and celebrated with an open house. The new floor expanded the space available for the family medicine, internal medicine, ophthalmology, otolaryngology, and patient education departments, making room for new practitioners and services. Drs. David Lundberg and Robert Jones, a new family practitioner with sports medicine training, opened a sports medicine service at the main clinic in June.

The Olmsted Medical Center explored ways to improve convenience and efficiency for patients, and a patient advocate was employed to assist patients with problems or concerns as part of the quality improvement system. A clinical pathway, or protocol, was established for obstetrical patients to streamline their management. An anticoagulation clinic was established to more efficiently serve patients taking blood-thinners and to improve their results. An advanced access system for appointments to reduce the wait time for visits to the primary care departments was implemented. The Olmsted Medical Center management initiated discussions with InteGreat Systems regarding installation of an electronic medical record system. Increased emphasis was placed on quality improvement in a variety of areas, and in October, the Olmsted Medical Center received an award from HealthPartners for its preventive care initiatives.

In September 2000, the public health department moved to its new building, and the Olmsted Medical Center began remodeling the health department offices in the hospital to accommodate the obstetrics and gynecology clinic. The exam rooms near the emergency department were converted for a future urgent care center. Having the obstetricians move to the hospital improved their efficiency in delivering patient care, since their outpatient exam rooms were located a minute or two from the obstetrics ward. The entrance for the health department on the north side of the hospital once again became the front entrance of the hospital. To improve services in Pine Island, ground was broken in November for a new, larger clinic there. A Christmas-morning fire destroyed the Wanamingo clinic, forcing the medical staff to move into temporary quarters in early 2002.

A consultant was engaged to assist the Olmsted Medical Center with one of the biggest issues it had had over the years: where and how large to build facilities to accommodate the growing numbers of patients and clinicians. One of the major questions was whether to consolidate the main clinic and the hospital at one location as we had hoped to do. But the projected costs of that option appeared to be prohibitive. After much discussion, a decision was made to maintain two campuses and to proceed with detailed planning for an expansion at the present hospital site.

The consultant's survey indicated that there was considerable interest among the respondents in starting a charitable foundation. The previous foundation of the Olmsted Medical Group had been dissolved several years earlier; and a new organization named the OMC Regional Foundation was established in the late summer of 2001. Its board of directors, led by Nancy Domaille as chair, held its first meeting in November. Other directors were Paul Barton, Jane Campion, Mr. Cartney, Hal Henderson, Greg House, Leigh Johnson, Dr. Pesch, Augie Schleicher, and, ex officio, Dan Berndt, Dr. Peterson, and Mr. Pitzer. The presence of an active foundation brought for the first time the opportunity to employ philanthropic support for some of the Olmsted Medical Center's frequent building projects and other activities. The Olmsted Medical Center had received some significant charitable donations even before the foundation was established. For example, Carl Petersen donated $50,000 in memory of his wife, Ihla. Mr. Petersen went on to leave a large part of his estate to the OMC Regional Foundation in trust, with the investment earnings to be used for providing medical care to needy residents of Olmsted County. The success of the Carl and Ihla Petersen Trust in assisting patients of the Olmsted Medical Center has inspired employees and others to contribute to the fund.

In May 2001, the Olmsted Medical Center joined the Institute for Clinical Systems Improvement (ICSI), a Twin-Cities-based organization that has become a national leader in developing practice guidelines and improving patient care. Olmsted Medical Center physicians and quality improvement personnel developed close working relationships with the ICSI staff, energizing our quality improvement projects. Although the Olmsted Medical Center benefited greatly from this association, the benefits came at a cost: Dr. Gary Oftedahl, our medical director, announced in November that he was leaving the Olmsted Medical Center after 25 years to become ICSI's medical director.

Implementation of an electronic medical record system had begun in May 2001, with the first departments online by August. All departments and physicians were using this system by early 2002. This was a huge advance because there were no more lost charts; chart creation, storage and retrieval costs were reduced; information was simultaneously available in all Olmsted Medical Center locations; and laboratory and radiology reports were loaded directly into the electronic record and could not be miscopied, misplaced, or lost. A prescription module permitted sending prescriptions directly by computer to pharmacies, avoiding the problem of indecipherable handwriting and ensuring complete documentation of medication orders in the record. The electronic prescription system later proved its worth with the recall of the anti-inflammatory drug Vioxx in 2004. Several hundred patients who had obtained prescriptions for the drug from Olmsted Medical Center physicians were easily identified and notified of the recall, a task that would have been practically impossible without an electronic medical record and drug prescribing system.

When a third general surgeon joined the Olmsted Medical Center in 2002, I took advantage of his arrival to semi-retire, taking off two half-days a week, and with no night call. I had agreed to become chairman of the Minnesota Medical Association board of trustees in September and was vice-chairman of the Midwest Medical Insurance Company. I finished my last night on call at 6:00 AM on January 2, 2002, the day the new surgeon started. At 7:00 PM, I received a call from the MMIC chairman, saying that he had to resign, and "Congratulations!" My semi-retirement lasted all of 13 hours.

Efforts to provide adequate space for clinical services continued into 2002, and the Olmsted Medical Center was fortunate to receive valuable assistance from local communities in which branch clinics were located. In Wanamingo, the local development group planned a new building across the street from the burned office to house the clinic and other offices, to open the following summer. The city of St. Charles proposed a building site for a new, larger clinic near the assisted-living facility in the northwest part of town. More space was leased to expand the Stewartville clinic. The Preston branch clinic, which was very busy already, came under increasing pressure when Dr. Sauer retired from his practice and the Gundersen Clinic reduced its services in nearby Harmony.

In spite of several years of concerted effort, the Hayfield clinic closed in December 2002 because of staffing problems, the long distance from Rochester, and lack of patient volume to meet basic expenses. It became apparent to the Olmsted Medical Center that branch clinics with only one doctor would not be financially feasible because of the large fixed overhead costs. Adding a second physician required only one additional medical assistant and about 20% more space, markedly reducing the cost per doctor.

As demands for detailed hospital discharge planning increased, a social services department was established, with Tricia Schilling employed as the hospital's first social worker. The service has since expanded to two social workers, who provide assistance to both outpatients and inpatients. The perinatal loss committee established the Still Missed Garden to further assist patients and others with their emotional needs. The garden is designed for patients, families, or staff of the Olmsted Medical Center who have experienced a loss. It is a place to plant an annual flower or plant in remembrance of loved ones, no matter what age, a place to gather and reflect, to honor and recognize the memories of loved ones.

With Dr. Oftedahl's departure to ICSI, the board decided to recruit a full-time chief medical officer, and Dr. David Westgard accepted the position in June 2002. A graduate of the University of Washington School of Medicine, Dr. Westgard completed a family medicine residency in San Bernardino, California. After service in the Air Force, he practiced at the Skemp Grandview Clinic in La Crosse for 23 years. Most recently, he had been chief medical officer at Shannon Health Systems in San Angelo, Texas. Dr. Westgard brought increased expertise in quality improvement and physician management and implemented changes in department chair functions and medical staff policies that have had long-lasting benefit.

Convenient patient access, a long-standing goal of the Olmsted Medical Center, was greatly improved when another new service, an urgent care department, opened at the hospital in March 2002. The urgent care staff was soon seeing an average of 72 patients per day, about double the expected volume, and with little impact on the emergency department's case load. In addition to improving access to its health services, the Olmsted Medical Center continued to invest heavily in medical technology, with upgrades to the CT and MRI scanners and to the ultrasound unit. The new technologies produced better images at higher speeds, thus increasing capacity.

By February 2003, the hospital expansion plans were complete. An addition would be built on the back of the hospital to increase the space for same-day surgery and other outpatient procedures and to create two new operating rooms. Below, on the first floor, the cafeteria would be enlarged, and in the basement a new, larger central sterile processing unit would be built. The move of the obstetricians to the hospital proved to be very successful, prompting consideration of moving the surgical departments to the hospital as well. It appeared that additional land would be needed for this, and the Olmsted Medical Center began to discuss with the city the possibility of acquiring the city maintenance garage property just west of the hospital to erect a building to house the surgical specialties. As noted previously, the state had sold this property to the county as part of the hospital building site, and the county had later given it to the city for the garage. The city of Rochester and the Olmsted Medical Center reached an agreement in 2005 for the Olmsted Medical Center to purchase and take possession of the property no later than 2012.

A momentous event occurred in September 2003, when the last of the hospital bonds were paid off two years early and the merger agreement with the county ended. The Olmsted Medical Center now owned the hospital outright, and the county commissioners no longer appointed five of the public trustees. The remaining trustees believed, however, that there was value in keeping some county representation among the public trustees. Two county commissioners completed their terms on the board and were replaced by Commissioners Jim Bier and Ken Brown. Mr. Devlin stayed on until the completion of his term in 2004. Throughout the duration of the agreement between the Olmsted Medical Center and the county commissioners, the relationship was cordial, collaborative, and constructive. Without the foresight of the county commissioners and their willingness to relinquish control of the hospital, the Olmsted Medical Center would not exist in its present form.

As the Olmsted Medical Center grew and matured, it began to receive recognition for its patient care, physicians, and operations. Solucient, an organization that evaluates hospitals for quality of care, efficiency of operations, and sustainability of performance, recognized the Olmsted Medical Center Hospital in 2003 as one of the top 100 hospitals in the country and one of the 20 best small community hospitals. The hospital also received special recognition from the Minnesota Department of Health for its improvements in skin care, reduction in patient falls, and marking surgical sites to avoid wrong-side surgery. Pediatrician Dr. Denise Bonde was awarded a prestigious Bush Foundation fellowship for additional study in allergy. Dr. Michael Mesick also received a Bush fellowship to study complementary and alternative medicine, including acupuncture, and both returned to the Olmsted Medical Center to practice. Dr. Barbara Yawn had become co-director of the Rochester Epidemiology Project the year before and was now named a member of the U.S. Preventive Services Task Force, a federal organization charged with making national recommendations for preventive care. She also served on the National Board of Medical Examiners and on panels for the National Institutes of Health.

The Olmsted Medical Center began voluntary participation with the Minnesota Community Measurement Project, which collects quality data from clinics for comparison and publication on the internet. The Olmsted Medical Center's performance on standard quality measures compared well to the scores of other organizations in Minnesota, and it received special mention for its accomplishments in hypertension care and cervical cancer screening.

Another changing of the guard occurred in 2006, when Dr. Roy Yawn replaced Dr. Peterson as president. Kevin Pitzer also left the position of chief administrative officer to return to Phoenix for another opportunity, and Tim Weir became the new chief administrative officer. Originally from Fargo, North Dakota, Mr. Weir had spent part of his career at the Fargo Clinic, but recently was vice president for the division of ambulatory services at

Bay State Health System in Springfield, Massachusetts. He is a graduate of the University of Minnesota and received a master's degree in healthcare administration and an MBA from the University of Iowa. In concert with the management staff, Mr. Weir has significantly strengthened the business operations and financial management of the Olmsted Medical Center.

The system of caring for hospitalized patients by physicians who rotated through the hospital service was replaced by a hospitalist program with full-time physicians whose only job is to manage the hospital patients. This system improves continuity of hospital care and adherence to hospital protocols and procedures. To improve patient safety, the hospital also implemented a rapid-response team at the hospital for patients with worsening conditions in order to avoid further deterioration or cardiac arrest. The hospital also implemented the "100,000 Lives" and "5,000,000 Lives" patient safety programs sponsored by the Institute for Healthcare Improvement.

In July 2006, the OMC Regional Foundation established the Dr. Noel R. Peterson Founders' Lecture series, funded by a generous gift from Dr. and Mrs. Peterson and supplemented by additional donations from friends and supporters of the foundation. This lecture series annually brings speakers to Rochester for a public address to the community about a variety of healthcare topics.

The hospital expansion and renovation was completed in December 2006. The new operating rooms, the expanded post-anesthesia recovery room, and the same-day surgery and outpatient procedures area were significant upgrades, and all the inpatient rooms were now private with showers. The less visible sterile processing unit in the basement of the addition was also a major improvement. A grand opening and Chamber of Commerce ribbon cutting was held on February 22, 2007.

With the proliferation of retail-based clinics and the likelihood that clinics of this type would come to Rochester, the board of governors authorized discussions with several businesses in Rochester in search of partners and likely sites. The board believed that this concept would be coming to the area in the near future, and thought that it would be a good service that the Olmsted Medical Center's patients desired. The board also strongly felt that such clinics should be part of the local healthcare system, directed and supervised by respected clinicians and with patient records that could be incorporated into the electronic medical record. The explorations led to a partnership with Bellin Health of Milwaukee and clinic locations in both Rochester Shopko stores.

The Olmsted Medical Center's first FastCare™ clinic opened in Rochester's north Shopko store July 16, 2007, becoming the first retail-based clinic in Rochester. The FastCare™ clinic at the south Shopko location opened on December 26, 2007. Nurse practitioners and physician assistants staff the clinics under the supervision of Drs. Michael Blue and Randy Hemann and with the assistance of Olmsted Medical Center specialists as needed. An important distinction from typical retail-based clinics is that these are part of the Olmsted Medical Center system, connected to the electronic medical records and with an ability to maintain continuity of care. The two clinics have been very successful and greatly appreciated by patients.

The radiology department implemented a $2.3 million project to convert all of the Olmsted Medical Center's imaging services to a digital system that would permit all images to be directly entered into the online medical record for viewing at all clinic locations. Conversion to a digital system eliminated the costs of X-ray films, processing with toxic chemicals, storage, and retrieval. The department also instituted a voice recognition dictation system for radiology reports, and the Olmsted Medical Center later added a similar system for all other dictated notes.

The Olmsted Medical Center opened a pathology department staffed by Dr. Durga Vege to supervise the laboratories and to perform surgical pathology and cytology, ending the 35-year supervisory arrangement with the Mayo Clinic department of pathology. Dr. Vege received her medical education and pathology training in India and was on the staff of the country's largest cancer center in Mumbai for 15 years. She came to the United States, retrained at the University of Minnesota and Regions Hospital in St. Paul, and worked in Winona for four years before joining the Olmsted Medical Center staff.

The year 2007 was a time of transitions for me. I finished my term on the Midwest Medical Insurance Company board in May, retired from surgery at the end of June, and completed the Minnesota Medical Association presidency in September. My time as board chair and president of Minnesota Medical Association was marked by a major push toward healthcare system redesign, which the association initiated with its Physicians' Plan for a Healthy Minnesota, the basis for much of the discussion about healthcare reform at the state legislature and the 2008 legislation, and by the state-wide ban on smoking in public places. Dr. Noel Peterson also played a major role in these processes and continues to be involved.

The Olmsted Medical Center has come a long way from Dr. Wente's tiny rented upstairs office 60 years ago and the promise of a community hospital—farther than anyone then ever dreamed. At the end of 2009, the Olmsted Medical Center's contribution to community benefits rose to more than $32 million. Its staff totaled 1,075, including 136 physicians and other clinicians. That year, more than 71,000 patients made about 280,000 visits. There were 3,320 hospital admissions totaling 8,023 patient days. There were 982 births and 3,608 surgical procedures. There were 32,732 emergency and urgent care visits and 27,596 visits to physical therapy.

To people from outside the Rochester area, it is shocking that the Olmsted Medical Center could grow to such a size in the same town as the world-famous Mayo Clinic. Almost inevitably, such a discussion will include the words "in the shadow of the Mayo Clinic." But today, the Olmsted Medical Center proudly stands in its own light. It is a vigorous, progressive medical institution with excellent physicians and other clinicians, effective leadership, modern medical technology and facilities, thousands of loyal patients, and support from the communities it serves. It is a high-quality healthcare organization with a bright future.

Chapter 12
Looking Back, and Forward

So, what lessons have we learned? How do we explain the amazing success of the Olmsted Medical Center? How did the Olmsted Medical Center get to be the way it is?

In the beginning, there were needs. As the Mayo Clinic became more specialized and subspecialized, there was a need for primary care physicians. The closed-staff hospitals of the Mayo Clinic discouraged other primary care physicians from coming to Rochester. Thus, to attract and retain primary care physicians, there was a need for a hospital they could use. There were other prominent needs also: the need for specialists to make the Olmsted Community Hospital succeed; the need for the Olmsted Medical Group to expand its services to keep the hospital viable; and the need for a unified, efficient, and effective healthcare system to meet the needs of a growing Rochester community and the surrounding area.

There were capable and visionary leaders who recognized the needs and pushed to meet them, in particular Dr. William F. Braasch, who worked tirelessly to establish the Olmsted Community Hospital and served on the board most of the remainder of his life; and Dr. Harold A. Wente, who led the development of the Olmsted Medical Group with vision, wisdom, and foresight, shaping its organization and culture. He was often on the leading edge of clinic development and sometimes a decade or two ahead in his vision of healthcare delivery. The organization and culture he established made it easy for his successors to continue on a path that sometimes seemed foreordained.

Capable administrators have also been a factor in the Olmsted Medical Center's success, and it has been fortunate to attract highly qualified people for those positions. Broad support from the public has also been important, too, from concerned citizens who led efforts to pass the referenda and voters who cast favorable ballots, to helpful legislators and county commissioners, to public advisory committee members, public trustees, and foundation board members who have given generously of their time and money.

The centralized governance structure started by Dr. Wente allowed timely decision-making and implementation. This permitted the Olmsted Medical Group and later the Olmsted Medical Center to be opportunistic and aggressive in meeting needs as they arose. As important as leadership has been the willingness of others to follow. The Olmsted Medical Group's physicians took the long-term view and supported unanimously or nearly so a series of decisions that strengthened the organization, sometimes against their own individual short-term interests.

The Olmsted Medical Center also had a rare willingness to invest in itself. In the last 20 years, hundreds or perhaps thousands of physician practices have been bought out by hospital chains, for-profit companies, and others because the doctors had been unwilling to invest in themselves and to accumulate the capital necessary to build modern practices. Today, thousands of physicians wait for the government or insurers to give them an electronic medical record, while successful groups like the Olmsted Medical Center and its patients have been benefiting from this technology for years.

The Olmsted Medical Center has excellent neighbors. The Mayo Clinic leadership encouraged both Dr. Braasch and Dr. Wente. While there have been occasional disagreements, the relationship, both on an institutional and a physician-to-physician level, has been exemplary, cooperative, and collaborative. In many other communities where there are competing group practices, the relationships are anything but cordial. The Mayo Clinic goes to great lengths to assist the Olmsted Medical Center in providing excellent care to all of its patients and to support its physicians and other clinicians with continuing medical education. The Mayo Clinic has welcomed Olmsted Medical Center physicians to its conferences and library, and has provided easy formal and informal consultations. Mayo Clinic doctors also have supported and encouraged Olmsted Medical Center physicians to participate in other medical organizations, such as the Minnesota Medical Association. Competition has made both organizations perform at a higher level than they might otherwise have. Our competition is aimed at trying to outdo one another in the quality of our patient services.

The Olmsted Medical Center has also enjoyed the cooperation and support of the Rochester city council, city administration, and the Olmsted County commissioners. The county's decision to merge the Olmsted Community Hospital with the Olmsted Medical Group and to cede control of the hospital to a private nonprofit organization was not easy. But it has proved to be beneficial to the citizens of Olmsted County and a large area of Southeastern Minnesota.

The Olmsted Medical Center's size and culture are good not only for patients; they also make it a great place to work. One of my patients a few years ago was a retired nurse from California who moved to Rochester to be near her daughter. When I saw her after her surgery, she commented at length about what a great hospital we had and how nice everyone was, things that I heard all the time. Then she said, "Do you know what I liked the best? The laughter. I heard so much laughing. It was obvious that everyone liked each other and enjoyed working together." It's true. We may be professionals, but we have fun, too. My co-workers made it worth getting up every morning for 33 years. A result of our pleasant work environment is that the Olmsted Medical Center has lower turnover rates than most medical centers and has many very long-term staff members. In May 2009, the Olmsted Medical Center celebrated the 50th anniversary of the employment of Shirley Young. Dr. Neal Olson recently surpassed Dr. Tom Peyla to hold the record among Olmsted Medical Center physicians for longevity at more than 41 years. About 10% of the staff are part of families that have two or more relatives working together at the Olmsted Medical Center. There is at least one three-generation family, spanning almost the entire hospital history. Kathy Haen, LPN, started at the Olmsted Community Hospital in the fall of 1955 and, with time out for children, worked until 1995. Her daughter, Kristi Ristau, RN, has been at the hospital since 1983, and another daughter, Colleen Burbank, LPN, started at the Olmsted Medical Group in 1991. Two granddaughters, Kaila Burbank and Christal Haen, began work at the hospital in 2005.

There continues and will continue to be a need for the Olmsted Medical Center. It has a sound structure and strong leadership, and it will develop or find capable future leaders who will continue to be attentive to the needs and opportunities to serve the Olmsted Medical Center's patients and communities. The Olmsted Medical Center's culture continues to reinforce itself and to work to improve patient care. Recently, more than one thousand staff members took part in advanced customer service training, building on past training and experience.

Providers of healthcare will continue to be under financial and regulatory pressure for the foreseeable future as the demand for healthcare far exceeds the resources to pay for it. The Olmsted Medical Center is well positioned to continue to survive times of stress as it stays true to its mission, vision, and core values.

Appendix A

Roster of Olmsted Medical Group and Olmsted Medical Center
Physicians, Podiatrists, and Psychologists

Clinician	Specialty	Tenure
Harold A. Wente	General Practice/Family Practice	1949-1987
James A. Doyle	General Practice/Obstetrics	1952-1979
John Stransky	General Practice	1953-1954
John (Jack) Verby	General Practice	1954-1968
John Watson	Obstetrics & Gynecology	1955-1959
Mary Price Pougiales	Ophthalmology	1955-1983
Harry Burich	Surgery	1955-1982
Beryl Kirklin	Radiology	1955-1957
Joe Teynor	General Practice	1956-1957
John Flanary	General Practice	1956-1958
Mary Obert	Internal Medicine	1956-1957
Malcolm Campbell	Internal Medicine	1956-1990
William Weyrauch	Surgery	1956-1959
John Brodhun	General Practice/Family Practice	1956-1993
Lloyd Wood	General Practice	1958-1963
John Fluegel	General Practice	1958-1966
John Garman	General Practice	1958-1959
Werner Kaese	Obstetrics & Gynecology	1959-1994
Frank V. Sander	Surgery	1961-1982
Clayton Bennett	General Practice/Family Practice	1962-1982
Charles (Chuck) Field	Obstetrics & Gynecology	1962-1969
James Hartfield	Pediatrics	1964-1985
Thomas Peyla	Pediatrics	1964-2006
Frederick Banfield	General Practice/Family Practice	1965-1980
James Garber	Internal Medicine	1967-2001
Neal Olson	Pediatrics	1968-
Robert Konicek	General Practice/Family Practice	1968-1990
Robert Rivan	Obstetrics & Gynecology	1969-1976
Sergio Grossling	Surgery	1970-1970
Nancy Grubbs	General Practice/Family Practice	1970-1981
Richard Christiana	General Practice/Family Practice	1970-
Larry Grubbs	General Practice/Family Practice	1970-2004
Thomas T. Myers	Vein Surgery	1972-1980

Sally Schneider	Obstetrics & Gynecology	1972-1976
James Beck	Internal Medicine	1972-1975
Cyril Corrigan	Radiology	1972-1989
Dale Hawk	General Practice St. Charles	1972-1974
Waldo Munderowski	General Practice St. Charles	1973-1973
Eugene Madsen	General Practice St. Charles	1973-1974
Patricia Connell	Family Practice	1973-1977
Allan Korn	General Practice	1974-1975
G. Richard Geier	Surgery	1974-2007
Mary Ann Kimmel (McNeilus)	General Practice	1974-1980
James Aquilino	Family Practice	1975-1977
Ingrid V. Neel	Pediatrics/Allergy	1975-2008
Margaret (Maggie) Fontana	Obstetrics & Gynecology	1976-1989
Gary L. Oftedahl	Internal Medicine	1976-2002
Rosalina Abboud	Obstetrics & Gynecology	1976-1991
Lee Chumbley	Ophthalmology	1976-1977
Dwain Stone	General Practice	1977-1980
Linda Butterfield	Ophthalmology	1979-2008
William Moravec	Obstetrics & Gynecology	1980-1983
Thomas Able	Family Practice	1980-1986
David Dillman	Ophthalmology	1980-1981
Kenneth Ubben	Dermatology	1981-1992
Jeff Morgan	Family Practice	1982-1989
Jeanne Mohler	Family Practice	1982-1991
Dennis Gannon	Psychology	1982-
Craig Thauwald	Family Practice Stewartville	1983-
Charles D. Branch	Surgery	1983-
Tim Keay	Family Practice	1983-1985
Joel Thompson	Family Practice	1983-1984
Elliott Eisenberg	Ophthalmology	1983-1984
Donald Ristad	Ophthalmology	1983-1984
Shirley Kunkel	Obstetrics & Gynecology	1983-1989
Noralane Lindor	Family Practice	1983-1991
Duane Ollendick	Psychology	1983-
Cynthia Bullen	Ophthalmology	1984-1985
Mark Stenberg	Internal Medicine	1984-
Harlan Wickre	Psychology	1985-
David Wall	Obstetrics & Gynecology	1985-2000

Roxolana Demczuk	Anesthesiology	1985-1986
Allan Clark	Family Practice Pine Island	1986-
Robert Nesheim	Psychiatry	1986-1989
J. Peter Frechette	Orthopedics	1986-1990
Beth Karon	Internal Medicine	1986-2002
Nora Hagen	Family Practice Stewartville	1986-1987
John Knight	Family Practice	1986-1987
Robert Grill	Ophthalmology	1986-
Allan Bakke	Anesthesiology	1986-2002
Denise Bonde	Pediatrics	1986-
Dale Hawk	Family Practice St. Charles	1986-1988
John Balkins	Family Practice St. Charles	1986-1997
Glenn Johnson	Orthopedics	1987-1989
Robert Breitenbach	Family Practice	1987-1991
Theresa Jensen	Family Practice	1987-1991
Bernard Matthieu	Family Practice Hayfield	1987-1988
Terri Edwards	Pediatrics	1987-
Loring Stead	Podiatry	1987-
Roland Matson	Family Practice Spring Valley	1987-1993
Brad Westra	Family Practice Spring Valley	1987-1997
Lynn Price	Family Practice	1988-1990
Daniel Pesch	Family Practice Elgin/Plainview	1988-
Kelli Leland	Family Practice Byron	1988-1989
Linda Williams	Family Practice Chatfield	1988-
Michelle Hanson	Family Practice St. Charles	1988-1989
Steve Vogel	Family Practice Hayfield	1988-2003
Christine Depenthal	Internal Medicine	1988-1993
Paula Chantigian	Obstetrics & Gynecology	1989-1991
Karen Lundquist	Radiology	1989-2002
Noel Peterson	Urology	1989-
Randy Hemann	Family Practice	1989-
Robert Kurland	Orthopedics	1989-
Thomas Erbach	Otolaryngology	1989-
Katherine Kainz	Psychology	1989-
Myron Kaminsky	Podiatry	1989-
Ruth Moes	Anesthesiology	1989-2001
Tony Santamaria	Anesthesiology	1989-
Lawrence Peterson	Psychiatry	1990-
Steve Henke	Family Practice Chatfield/Preston	1990-2003

Nancy Peltola	Family Practice St. Charles/Preston	1990-2003
Craig Chambers	Internal Medicine	1990-
Roy Yawn	Internal Medicine	1990-
Thomas Miller	Family Practice	1990-
Thomas McGuffin	Radiology	1990-2009
Doris Lin	Family Practice Byron	1990-1998
Annette Krutsch	Psychology	1990-2000
Robert Sookochoff	Family Practice Spring Valley	1990-1993
Glenn Faith	Emergency Medicine	1990-1992
James Smith	Neurology	1991-
Shelly Giebel	Obstetrics & Gynecology	1991-1994
Peter Arndt	Pediatrics	1991-
Hila McCoy	Pediatrics	1991-
Heather Bevan	Family Practice	1991-1993
Robert Reed	Family Practice Byron	1991-1993
Steven Harder	Family Practice Spring Valley	1991-
Raymond Krueger	Family Practice Spring Valley	1992-
David Lundberg	Family Practice	1992-
Barbara Yawn	Research	1992-
Rose Christian	Internal Medicine	1992-1996
Gail Knops	Family Practice	1992-1994
Nancy Fazekas	Family Practice Pine Island	1992-1994
David Handley	Emergency Medicine	1992-
Jeff McNally	Emergency Medicine	1992-1993
Isaac Yoon	Acute Illness	1992-1998
Kim Kramer McKeon	Obstetrics & Gynecology	1992-
Kathy Hoyer	Family Practice Stewartville	1992-2002
Boris Velkov	Obstetrics & Gynecology	1993-2001
Louis Wagner	Radiology	1993-
Rick Kvam	Emergency Medicine	1993-
Shaun Dekutoski	Family Practice Byron	1993-
Paul Malinda	Emergency Medicine	1993-1996
Mary Beer	Psychology	1993-
Raymond DeLorenzi	Orthopedics	1994-1999
Kathryn Lombardo	Psychiatry	1994-
Martha Bowman	Internal Medicine	1994-
Michael Mesick	Family Practice Chatfield	1994-
Sam Minor	Family Practice Hayfield	1994-1996
B.J. Morrill	Family Practice	1994-1996

James Hoffmann	Obstetrics & Gynecology	1994-
Adele Moreland	Dermatology	1994-1999
Stephanie Jakim	Family Practice Preston	1994-
Charles Slater	Family Practice Spring Valley	1994-
Timothy Hunter	Family Practice	1994-1997
Ruth Archibald	Family Practice Pine Island	1994-1997
Brid MacBride	Family Practice Northwest	1995-2007
Cassandra Harrison	Emergency Medicine	1996-1999
Deborah Villenueve	Obstetrics & Gynecology	1996-1998
John Cierzan	Internal Medicine	1996-
Jane Cooper	Internal Medicine	1997-
Kristin Arndt	Pediatrics	1997-
Bobbi Kostinek	Family Practice Pine Island	1997-2005
Victoria Dietz	Family Practice	1997-
Victoria Hagstrom	Family Practice St. Charles	1997-2006
Todd Wade	Family Practice Northwest	1998-2002
Charles Dicken	Dermatology	1998-2005
Mark James	Radiology	1998-2005
Carole Nistler	Family Practice	1998-
Marlys Christianson	Family Practice	1998-2003
Mary Evans	Obstetrics & Gynecology	1998-2001
Harry Swedlund	Allergy	1998-2003
Timothy Gabrielson	Orthopedics	1999-2006
Pam Mergens	Anesthesiology	1999-2000
Dawn Allison	Dermatology	1999-2000
Coco Dughi	Internal Medicine	1999-2003
Afzal Ammar	Internal Medicine	1999-2005
Lindy Hankel	Internal Medicine St. Charles	1999-
Julie Chen	Family Practice	1999-2001
Barry Barudin	Pediatrics	1999-2003
Sean Gupton	Emergency Medicine	1999-2000
Robert Jones	Family Practice	2000-2008
Robert Merrill	Family Practice	2000-
Lon Krieg	Family Practice Hayfield	2000-2002
Kristen Bergstrom	Emergency Medicine	2000-2004
Jay Myers	Emergency Medicine	2000-
James Baber	Anesthesiology	2000-
Lissa Dias Ecker	Obstetrics & Gynecology	2000-2004
Hyeon Choi	Pediatrics	2000-2004

Jeffrey Gursky	Psychiatry	2000-
Kevin Weber	Psychology	2000-
Srdan Babovic	Plastic Surgery	2001-
Robert Fischer	Obstetrics & Gynecology	2001-2003
Dae Yang	Emergency Medicine	2001-
Sean O'Grady	Urgent Care	2001-2006
Barbara Loring	Psychology	2001-
Eric Etzel	Anesthesiology	2001-2004
Sharon Hargraves	Anesthesiology	2001-2002
Michael Migden	Dermatology	2001-2002
Dwain Stone	Surgery	2002-2003
Jaroslaw Aniszewski	Internal Medicine	2002-2005
James Killian	Radiology	2002-2004
David E. Westgard	Family Practice, Chief Medical Officer	2002-
Sharon Libi	Otolaryngology	2002-
David Lowe	Allergy	2002-
Aimee Perri	Pediatrics	2002-2006
Joseph Tricario	Anesthesiology	2002-
Jill Abramson	Pediatrics/Research	2002-2003
Lizzie Giangreco	Obstetrics & Gynecology	2002-2003
Andrew Jacobson	Family Practice Stewartville	2002-2003
Jae Lee	Family Practice Northwest	2002-2003
Patience Owan	Pediatrics	2003-2007
Kristen Hanzel	Internal Medicine	2003-2005
John Knight	Family Practice Byron	2003-2005
Dale Loeffler	Family Practice Preston	2003-
Margaret North	Dermatology	2003-
Diya Odeh	Radiology	2003-
Richard Peirce	Anesthesiology	2003-2009
Dane Treat	Family Practice	2003-2005
Wendy White	Obstetrics & Gynecology	2003-2009
Kathleen Frekko	Internal Medicine	2003-2004
Vidhan Chandra	Surgery	2004-
Duane Bartels	Family Practice	2004-
Patricia Cackowski	Family Practice Stewartville	2004-2009
Indrani Chaudry	Pediatrics	2004-
Leah Holmgren	Internal Medicine	2004-2007
Jack Perrone	Obstetrics & Gynecology	2004-

Andrea Jolley	Emergency Medicine	2004-2005
Therese Zink	Family Practice/Research	2004-2006
Mario Potvin	Surgery	2005-
Kathy Bonapace	Obstetrics & Gynecology	2005-2006
Peter Anagnostopoulis	Emergency Medicine	2005-
Jon Van Loon	Psychiatry	2005-
Michael Blue	Family Practice Wanamingo	2005-
Kirby Clark	Radiology	2005-2009
Barbara Backer	Internal Medicine	2005-2007
Leah Holmgren	Internal Medicine	2005-2007
Prasamsi Mikkelineni	Internal Medicine	2005-
Melanie Johnson	Family Practice	2005-
Dan Swartz	Family Practice Northwest	2005-
Mark Wilbur	Family Practice Byron	2005-
Arjun Bamzai	Pediatrics	2005-
Thomas Matzke	Dermatology	2005-2006
Eve Berryhill	Psychiatry	2006-
Brian Jacobs	Family Practice Pine Island	2006-209
Cathryn Silver	Psychology	2006-2008
Paulo Guimaraes	Hospital Medicine	2006-
Durga Vege	Pathology	2007-
Carol Kosmicke	Psychiatry	2007-
Louise Del Paine	Radiology	2007-2008
Karen Chen	Dermatology	2007-
Suzanne Pfeffer-Kleeman	Anesthesiology	2007-
Amy Larson	Internal Medicine	2007-
Claude Bridges	Hospital Medicine	2007-
Aaron Hanesworth	Family Practice St. Charles	2007-2010
Vicky Hagstrom	Family Practice Northwest	2007-2009
Deepika Bhargava	Pediatrics	2008-
Tina Hahn	Pediatrics	2008-
Brenda Brown	Family Practice	2008-
Kenneth Palmer	Obstetrics & Gynecology	2008-
Ehab Michael	Internal Medicine	2008-
Joel Solano	Ophthalmology	2008-
Jeff Beckenbaugh	Orthopedics	2008-
Amy Burns	Pediatric Anesthesia	2008-
Michel Barsoum	Hospital Medicine	2008-
Malik Al-Omari	Hospital Medicine	2008-

Patricia Aguedelo-Suarez	Obstetrics & Gynecology	2008-
Marcia Guerten	Psychology	2009-
Jessica Flynn	Family Practice Pine Island	2009-
Bhuma Srinivasan	Endocrinology	2009-
David Morrell	Radiology	2009-
Matt Thompson	Sports Medicine	2009-
Tamara Alexandrov	Orthopedics	2009-
Elizabeth McDonald	Radiology	2009-
William Wells	Radiology	2009-

Index

Abboud, Rosalina, MD, 80

Abboud, Mark, 96

Affeldt, D.E., MD, 37

Ahmann, Rosemary, 88, 90

Allen, John W., 93-96, 99, 103

Allen, W.A., MD, 14-15

Alvarez, Walter C., MD, 39

Anderson, Ron, 128

Aquilino, James, MD, 77, 78

Baars, C.W., MD, 63

Bakke, Allan, MD, 133

Balcombe, John L., MD, 7

Balkins, John, MD, 133

Banfield, Fred, MD, 86, 90, 101

Bardwell, Ira C., MD, 8, 9

Barton, Paul, 172

Bendzick, Robert, 141

Bennett, Clayton, MD, 52, 54, 57, 109

Berg, Tom, 108

Bergsland, Tom, 149, 157, 164

Berkowitz, Eric, PhD, 105, 108, 109, 147

Berndt, Dan, 157, 164, 172

Betcher, Craig, 94

Bianco, Anthony, MD, 26

Bier, Jim, 175

Birdseye, Art, 90

Blue, Michael, MD, 178

Bohmbach, Julia Marchant, RN, 3, 39, 87

Bonde, Denise, MD, 176

Booth, Alane, PA, 169

Booth, Norman, PA, 165

Bowman, Martha, MD, 159, 160

Braasch, William F., MD, 3, 17-19, 23, 31-39, 46-48, 181, 182

Bradley, Rep. Fran, 162

Branch, Charles D., MD, 109, 110, 136, 150, 164, 166, 169

Brandt, Robert, 127, 130, 131, 139

Brataas, Sen. Nancy, 90

Brezicka, Karen Wheelock, RN, MSN, 140, 164

Brodhun, John, MD, 44, 54, 101, 109, 112, 123, 171

Bromberg, Robert, 144, 149, 154, 156, 157

Brown, Ken, 175

Brunsgaard, James E., 84-87, 91, 92

Buenger, E.W., 33, 34

Buie, Louis, MD, 46

Bundy, Glenn, 38

Burbank, Colleen, LPN, 183

Burbank, Kaila, 183

Burich, Harry F., MD, 36, 37, 42, 44, 48-54, 59, 73, 101, 104, 107, 109, 125

Butterfield, Joseph, MD, 104

Butterfield, Linda, MD, 104

Campbell, Malcolm, MD, 43, 44, 52, 54, 57, 123

Campion, Jane, 172

Cannady, James A., 2, 39, 84,

Canney, Joseph, 133

Carlson, Gov. Arne, 162

Carlsson, Ed, PhD, 111

Cartney, Joe, 87, 140, 149, 153, 154, 161, 164, 172

Chambers, Craig, MD, 152

Chase, Richard, 93

Christiana, Richard, MD, 63, 84

Cierzan, John, MD, 160

Clark, Allan, MD, 129

Cooper, Charles C., MD, 39

Corrigan, Cyril, MD, 41, 63, 64, 67

Crewe, John E., MD, 16, 17

Cross, Edwin Childs, MD, 8-12, 15, 16, 27

Cross, Elisha Wild, MD, 8-12

Cross, J. A. Grosvenor, MD, 15, 16

Cunningham, Kevin, CRNA, 2

Cunningham, Rita, 2

Cysewski, Irene, RN, 34

Daly, Joe, 23

Davenport, Lance, 149, 152, 157, 164

Davids, Rep. Greg, 162

Davis, Noreen, RN, 94, 96, 131, 135, 139, 140

Daywitt, Francis "Shorty", 39

DeLorme, Connie, PhD, 73

Demczuk, Roxolana, MD, 129, 133

Devlin, Richard, 3, 84, 89, 141, 142, 161, 164, 175

Dicken, Charles, MD, 67

Domaille, Nancy, 172

Dougherty, Guy, 77, 78

Doyle, James A., MD, 26-29, 35, 37, 50-54, 80, 104

Doyle, Mary, 26, 45

Eckstrand, Leonard, 18, 37

Ellis, E.W., MD, 37, 48, 106

Etbauer, Dennis, 133, 151, 164, 165

Eusterman, Matthew, DDS, 46

Evenson, T.G., DDS, 19, 31

Feldman, F.M., MD, 17, 18

Ferguson, Thomas, 164

Field, Charles, MD, 53, 54, 62

Flanary, John, MD, 43, 45, 50

Fleming, Robert, 76, 78, 85, 89, 102, 103, 125

Fluegel, John, MD, 45, 48-51, 54

Fontana, Margaret, MD, 80

Frechette, Peter, MD, 132, 146

Freeman, Kit, 141

Friedrich, William, 47

Fuller, Ben, MD, 61

Gabrielson, Sharon, MSN, 167

Gahnstrom, Greg, 110

Galloway, Hector, MD, 8, 10, 12

Gannon, Dennis, 108, 110

Garber, James, MD, 59-62, 70, 78, 110, 149, 155, 156, 160

Gau, Coleen, RN, 73, 156

Geier, G. Richard, MD, 1-4, 71-74, 77, 80, 91-94, 96, 101, 104, 108, 109, 121, 123-126, 128-137, 139, 141-144, 146, 148, 150, 152-154, 156-160, 163, 164, 166, 167, 170, 173, 174, 178, 183

Geier, Karen, RN, 71-73

Gibbons, Stan, 64

Giese, O.P., 34

Glabe, R.A., 37

Gores, Robert, DDS, 98

Graham, Christopher, MD, 11, 15, 27

Granger, Charles T., MD, 14,15

Granger, Gertrude Booker , MD, 15

Granger, Pearl, 47

Grassle, Paul, 31, 34

Grill, Robert, MD, 133

Grubbs, Larry, MD, 62, 146

Grubbs, Nancy, MD, 62, 107

Gunsalas, Gwen, 127

Haen, Christal, 183

Haen, Kathy, LPN, 183

Hall, O.H., MD, 14

Hammarstad, Virgil, 134

Hanson, Stuart, MD, 165

Hargesheimer, Dick, 45

Hartfield, James, MD, 53, 54, 60, 70, 72, 85, 105, 124, 130

Hartfield, Sally, 72

Harwick, Harry, 23, 27, 42, 107

Hassett, Sr. Joyce, RN, 79

Hawk, Dale, MD, 63, 68, 69, 73, 133

Hemann, Randy, MD, 169, 178

Henderson, Hal, 165, 172

Herb, Isabella, MD, 15

Hettwer, Elaine Bassi, 131

Hodgson, John R., MD, 76, 78, 85, 86, 89

Holets, Thomas, MA, MBA, 105, 109, 124-129, 133-135, 141, 143-149, 154-159, 161, 164, 166

Holland, Cleon, MD, 49

Houglum, Arvid, MD, 140, 141

House, Greg, 172

Humphrey, Sen. Hubert H., 29, 42, 43

Hunt, James, MD, 78

Hunter, James, MD, 49

Huntley, Rep. Tom, 162

Jakim, Stephanie, MD, 160

Jenkins, Mark, 166, 167

Johnson, Glenn, MD, 146, 148

Johnson, Leigh, 172

Jones, James, 47

Jones, Robert, MD, 171

Joyce, George L., MD, 25, 37, 46

Joyce, George T., MD, 15

Kaese, Dottie, 51

Kaese, Werner, MD, 50, 51, 54, 69, 80, 123, 159

Kahler, John L., 16

Kamper, Carol, 86, 164

Katz, Hazel, 39

Keith, Norman, MD, 57

Keith, Sandy, 89-92, 139

Kelley, Lewis, MD, 8, 9

Kimmel, Mary Ann, MD, 78

Kirklin, Beryl, MD, 41, 185

Kiscaden, Sen. Sheila, 162

Klenner, Sue, RN, 131, 168

Konicek, Robert, MD, 60

Konicek, Trudy, 60

Krueger, Douglas, 93

Kuhlman, S.A., 47

Kurland, Leonard, MD, 57, 148

Kurland, Robert, MD, 148

Kurowski, James, MD, 142, 149, 151-155

Lindeman, Roger, MD, 165

Linville, Cedric, 35, 39, 46-49, 53, 67, 72, 74, 83, 85, 87

Lobb, A.J., 18, 31, 33

Lowrey, George, 27

Ludowese, Paul, 85

Lund, George, MD, 42

Lundberg, David, MD, 155, 171

Lundquist, Karen, MD, 153

Lundy, J.S., MD, 33

Maass, Henry T., 47

MacBride, Brid, MB, ChB, 156

Mahle, D.G., MD, 37

Marren, Dan, 167, 169

Matson, Roland, MD, 108, 133, 146

Mayberry, Eugene, MD, 86, 125

Mayo, Charles Horace, MD, 12-17, 27

Mayo, Charles W. "Chuck," MD, 9-13, 27

Mayo, William James, MD, 3, 13-17

Mayo, William Worrall, MD, 8-13

McHutchison, Sam, MD, 69

McKaig, C.B., MD, 37, 38

McLane, Barbara, 157

Melvin, Duane "Dewey," 47

Mesick, Michael, MD, 176

Meyers, Glenn, 91

Millett, Melvin C., MD, 15

Mills, Millard, 42, 55

Moes, Mother Alfred, 13

Mohler, Jeanne, MD, 107, 108

Mondale, Vice-president Walter, 103

Monson, Donald, 107

Morgan, Jeffrey, MD, 107, 130

Myers, Thomas T., MD, 67

Nagle, Karen, PhD, 157, 164

Neel, Bryan, MD, 79

Neel, Ingrid, MD, 79, 104, 123, 124

Nehring, John, MD, 148

Nelson, Doug, DDS, 45

Nelson, Terry, 164

Nesheim, Robert, MD, 132, 151

Nobrega, Fred, MD, 57

Obert, Mary, MD, 43

Ochsner, C.G., MD, 37

Oftedahl, Gary, MD, 80, 81, 94,
111, 123, 126, 128, 130, 155,
169, 173, 174

Olson, E.A., 37

Olson, Lynn, 99, 127

Olson, Neal, MD, 60, 74, 183

Orgel, David, MD, 167

O'Sullivan, Michael, MD, 68

Page, Ray, MD, 35, 37

Pagenhart, Clarence C., 27, 28

Pavlish, Charles, 146, 149, 157

Pemberton, John deJ., Jr., 34, 39

Perpich, Gov. Rudy, 90

Pesch, Daniel, MD, 169, 172

Petersen, Carl, 172, 173

Petersen, Ihla, 172, 173

Petersen, Magnus, MD, 33

Peterson, Larry, MD, 151, 169

Peterson, Noel, MD, 147, 148, 156,
169, 171, 172, 176, 177, 179

Peyla, Betty (Anderson), 53

Peyla, Thomas, MD, 53, 54, 60, 146,
156, 164, 169, 183

Pitzer, Kevin, 169, 172, 176

Platt, James, 144, 157

Plunkett, Richard, 28, 29, 42, 50, 52, 55

Plunkett, Warren, 42

Podulke, Michael, 164

Pougiales, George, 36

Pougiales, Mary (Price), MD, 36, 50,
54, 104

Preuhs, Dessa, RN, 87

Pruitt, Ray, MD, 77

Pudwell, Bill, 157, 164

Rian, Jim, 149

Riddick, Frank, MD, 165

Riggott, Brenda, 164

Risser, Alden, MD, 37, 47, 49, 52,
63, 68, 108, 160

Ristau, Kristy, RN, 183

Rivan, Robert, MD, 80

Rollins, Pat, MD, 37

Rossi, Dick, DDS, 45

Rubin, Leonard, MD, 80

Rueber, Joel, 3, 165

Ruegg, Russ, 38

Ruffalo, Carl, 64

Sabbann, Robert, DPM, 46

Salzman, Stan, 144

Sander, Frank V., MD, 51, 54, 73,
107, 109

Sauer, Robert, MD, 133, 148, 174

Schuett, Sue, 164

Schilling, Trisha, MSW, 174

Schlachter, Sandy, 169

Schleicher, Augie, 172

Schmitz, Ray, 141, 162

Schneider, Sally, MD, 80

Schrantz, Robert, MD, 67

Shuster, Slade, 23

Sitzer, Thomas, DDS, 157

Skaar, Robert, 49

Skaug, H.M., MD, 37

Slatterly, Calvin T., 47

Smith, James, MD, 150

Spring, Nicholas, 103

Stafford, Troy, 167

Stead, Loring, DPM, 170

Stenberg, Mark, MD, 149, 164, 170

Stewart, Howard "Chub", 140, 141

Stinchfield, Augustus W., MD, 15, 17

Stransky, John, MD, 29, 35

Swedlund, Harry, MD, 67

Taylor, William, MD, 140

Tews, Avery, 18, 31, 32

Teynor, Joe, MD, 43, 50

Thauwald, Craig, MD, 108, 141, 164

Thomforde, Larry, 105

Tiedeman, Gerald, 90

Till-Tarara, Lois, 164

Tinker, John, MD, 71

Tointon, Bill, 149

Tompkins, Dick, MD, 128

Truscott, Gerald D., 83, 84

Ubben, Kenneth, MD, 107

Utz, Virginia, RN, 39

Vege, Durga, MD, 178

Verby, John, MD, 35-37, 47,
    48-54, 57-61

Vihstadt, C.B., 17, 19

Watson, John, MD, 36, 37, 44, 50

Wellner, Ted, MD, 23-25, 37-39,
    46, 48, 63

Wente, Aloysious, 21

Wente, Elaine Daly, 22-24, 36, 38-41,
    50, 159, 160

Wente, Eugene, 21, 22

Wente, Harold Alois, MD, 2, 3, 21-29,
    31-39, 41-46, 49-57, 59-62, 65,
    67-73, 76-79, 90, 91, 101-104, 107,
    125, 126, 145, 147, 156, 158-160,
    179, 181, 182

Westgard, David, MD, 174

Westin, Harold, 58, 59, 134

Westra, Brad, MD, 133, 146

Weyhrauch, Bill, MD, 44, 50

Whisnant, Jack, MD, 57, 58

Weir, Tim, 177,

Wilkus, Frank J., 42, 44, 52-55, 57,
    69-73, 76, 78, 85, 90, 91, 102-105,
    107, 109-112, 124

Wilson, Viktor, MD, 31

Winholtz, Howard, 86

Wood, Lloyd, MD, 45, 50, 52

Yawn, Barbara, MD, 152-156, 166, 176

Yawn, Roy, MD, 152, 176

Young, Shirley, 183

Zubay, Rep. Kenneth, 90

General Index

"In the Shadow of the Shadow," 166

Accreditation Association for Ambulatory Health Care, 67, 112

Albert Lea Medical Group, 145

Ambulance service, 38, 39, 169

American Medical Group Association, 3, 61, 126

American Academy of Medical Directors, 70, 105, 128, 130

American Association of Medical Clinics, now AMGA, 61, 70

American College of Physician Executives, 70

American Group Practice Association, now AMGA, 70, 76, 126, 128, 144

Austin (Mn) Clinic, 70, 104

Baldwin building, 106, 148

Blue Cross, 48

Blue Cross and Blue Shield of Minnesota, 102, 104, 125, 134

Buffalo Wallow, 27, 33

Byron, 27, 91, 105, 146

Cascade Creek, 7

Cascade Rest and Milk Sanitarium, 16

Chatfield, 37, 93, 146, 149, 153, 160

Chute Sanitorium, 16

Citizens' Voluntary Hospital Committee, 18, 31

Cleveland Clinic, 29

College of American Pathologists, 169

Colonial Hospital, 16

Community BirthCenter, 97, 130, 139

Computerized Tomography (CT), 145, 148, 150, 151, 153–156, 167, 168, 175

Cook House, 16

CyCare, 150

Daybreak, 110, 125, 129, 130, 135, 139

Diagnosis Related Groups (DRGs), 97, 111, 131

Dodge Center, 78

Electronic medical record, 80, 150, 171, 173, 178, 182

Elgin, 37, 48, 106-108, 112, 146, 169

Ellerbe & Co., 32-34, 49, 55, 56

Employee Retirement Income and Security Act of 1974 (ERISA), 75

FastCare ™, 178

Flood, 27, 33, 89, 91, 92

Gundersen Clinic, 36, 80, 111, 151, 174

Hammel, Green and Abrahamson, 93, 165

Hayfield, 41, 70, 148, 149, 174

Health Maintenance Organizations (HMOs), 75, 76, 102, 103, 125, 128, 134, 135, 167

Health Systems Agencies (HSAs), 75, 103

HealthPartners, 167, 171

Hill-Burton funds, 32, 47, 48, 49, 56

Hillcrest, 50, 54-56, 59, 62, 65

HMO Minnesota, 102, 103, 135

IBM, 41, 44, 45, 65, 87, 91, 157, 167

Institute for Clinical Systems Improvement (ICSI), 173, 174

InteGreat Systems, 150, 171

Internal Revenue Service [IRS], 52, 125, 144, 154-157, 159, 165

Kahler House, 16

Kasson, 25, 37, 69, 77, 78

Lawler Building, 23, 26

Lutheran Brotherhood, 59, 124, 125, 134, 142

Magnetic Resonance Imaging (MRI), 167, 168, 175

Mayo Clinic, 3, 5-8, 14-18, 23-26, 28, 29, 31-36, 38-42, 44-46, 50-54, 57-63, 67-69, 72-74, 76-80, 85-89, 92, 102-107, 121, 125, 128, 129, 133, 134, 144, 145-155, 158, 165, 166, 168, 169, 178-182

Mayo Clinic Board of Governors, 19, 35, 86

Mayo Clinic pathology department, 68

Mayo Clinical Reviews, 36

Mayo family practice residency, 76-78

Mayo Health Plan, 135

Mayo Medical School, 68, 76-78, 129

Medical Economics, 5, 41, 42

Medical Properties, 28, 50

Medical Service, 56, 75, 123, 145, 171

Medicare, 75, 84, 87, 96, 97, 111, 112, 125, 126

Merger, 139- 143, 153, 159, 161-168, 175

Midwest Medical Insurance Company, MMIC Group, 160, 173, 178

Minnesota Department of Revenue, 165

Minnesota Medical Association, 156, 167, 173, 178, 182

Minnesota Department of Health, 32, 176

Minnesota State Legislature, 33, 52, 98, 179

Miracle Mile shopping center, 43

Ninth Street building, 124, 159

Non-profit, Not-for- profit, 76, 79, 156, 158

OCH Medical Staff, 37, 45-49, 53, 55-59, 63, 65, 74, 84, 86, 93, 94, 98, 127, 131, 136, 140, 153, 154, 157, 163

Ochsner Clinic, 29

Ochsner Medical Center, 165

Olmsted Community Hospital, 16, 34-39, 41, 45-47, 51-58, 63- 65, 67, 68, 69, 72, 74, 83-89, 91-99, 101-106, 110, 112, 127, 130, 131-135, 137, 139, 141, 142, 148-150, 153, 157-162, 164, 181-183

Olmsted Community Health Center, 17, 27, 31-33, 89, 153, 155, 157, 161

Olmsted Community Hospital Auxiliary, 3, 48, 63, 74, 92, 94, 95, 136, 165

Olmsted Community Hospital Board, 34, 35, 39, 46, 48, 49, 63, 65, 83-85, 91, 92, 98, 136, 139, 140, 149, 151, 153

Olmsted Community Hospital Foundation, 96

Olmsted County Board of Commissioners, 31, 86, 92, 162, 175, 176, 181, 182

Olmsted County Health Department, 17, 18, 83, 88, 90, 130, 136, 140-142, 153, 161, 168, 172

Olmsted Medical and Healthcare Foundation, 149

Olmsted Medical Group, 2, 3, 28, 29, 35-38, 41- 48, 50- 65, 67, 71, 75-78, 81-84, 98, 99, 101, 102-106, 110-112, 121, 123, 126, 128, 131, 132, 135, 136, 139, 141, 142, 145, 151, 152-158, 161-164, 172, 181-185

Olmsted Medical Properties, 124, 159

OMC Regional Foundation, 172, 177

OMG Northwest branch clinic, 149, 165, 166

OMG profit-sharing trust, 55, 56, 65, 107, 111, 124, 125

OMG Public Advisory Committee, 149, 156, 157 , 181

OMG, OMC Board of Governors, 152, 157, 164, 165, 168, 169, 177

OMG, OMC Board of Trustees, 157, 158, 162, 163, 168, 169

Optical shop, 64

Over the Rainbow, 141

Pine Island, 25, 37, 129, 133, 148, 149, 164, 172

Plainview, 14, 37, 41, 45, 106, 169

Rochester Post-Bulletin , Post-Bulletin, 3, 17-19, 28, 29, 31, 33, 41, 45, 47, 49, 69, 74, 84-99, 103, 104, 127, 139, 158, 162, 163

Preston, 108, 129, 133, 148, 160, 162, 174

Professional association, professional corporation, 52, 61, 144, 156, 158

Professional Services Review Organizations (PSROs), 75, 76

Referendum 1948, 19, 23, 31, 32, 34, 49

Referendum 1978, 88-93

Riverside Hospital, 14, 15

Rochester City Council, 13, 15, 32, 33, 38, 42, 159, 182

Rochester Epidemiology Project, 57, 61, 154, 176

Rochester Methodist Hospital, 16, 68, 83, 86- 89, 93, 101, 103, 148

Rochester State Hospital, 12, 53

Ruffalo Pharmacy, 50

Salk Polio vaccine, 37

Samaritan Bethany Nursing Home, 12, 16

Southeast Minnesota Health Systems Agency, 91, 78, 103

Sisters of St. Francis, 13

Smoking, 56, 62-65, 126, 179

Southeast Minnesota HMO, 102, 103

Southeast Minnesota HMO Consortium, 102, 103

Spring Valley, 108, 133, 146, 149

St. Louis Park Clinic, now Park-Nicollet Medical Center, 42, 64, 80

St. Charles, 35, 37, 43, 45, 63, 68, 69, 73, 133, 174

St. Marys Hospital, 13-17, 26, 28, 34, 38, 39, 68, 69, 83-89, 97, 151

Stewartville, 17, 18, 25, 34, 37, 39, 46, 68, 108, 112, 129, 133, 160, 174

Tax exemption, tax-exempt, 143, 144, 149, 153, 154, 157, 159, 161, 163, 165

The Joint Commission, 46, 74, 131, 164, 165, 169,

Third Avenue building, 53, 55, 56, 63, 88, 107, 124

U.S. Department of Labor, 75, 107, 111, 125

Under the Weather, 131, 136, 141

Van Dusen mansion, 27

Wanamingo, 165, 174

Zumbrota Clinic, 165

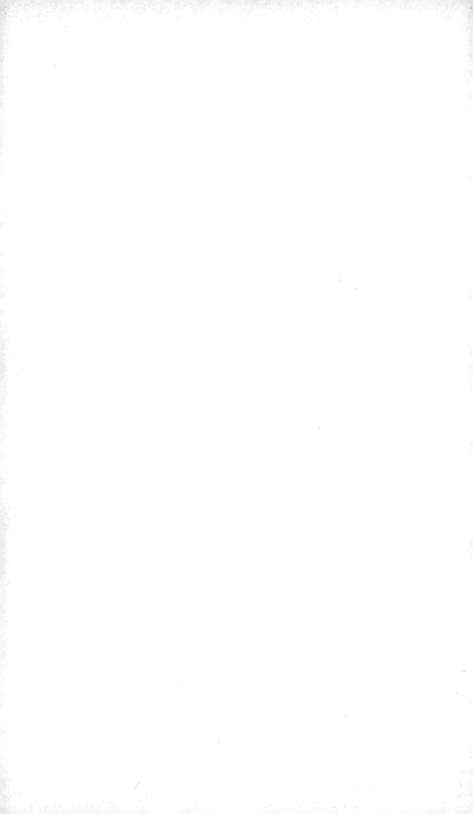